Introducing
Palliative Care

Fourth edition

Robert Twycross DM, FRCP, FRCR

Emeritus Clinical Reader in Palliative Medicine, Oxford University
Academic Director, Oxford International Centre for Palliative Care
Head, WHO Collaborating Centre for Palliative Care, Oxford, UK

RADCLIFFE MEDICAL PRESS

Radcliffe Medical Press Ltd
18 Marcham Road
Abingdon
Oxon OX14 1AA
United Kingdom

www.radcliffe-oxford.com
The Radcliffe Medical Press electronic catalogue and online ordering facility.
Direct sales to anywhere in the world.

First edition 1995
Second edition 1997
Third edition 1999

British Library Cataloguing in Publication Data

A catalogue record for this book is available from the British Library.

ISBN 1 85775 915 X

Typeset by Advance Typesetting Ltd, Oxon
Printed and bound by TJ International Ltd, Padstow, Cornwall

Contents

Preface

Introducing Palliative Care is the manual for several foundation courses run in Oxford, India and elsewhere. I hope that others will find it of value and use it in a similar way. In this fourth edition, the focus of *Introducing Palliative Care* is still on the care of patients with advanced cancer. However, the general principles and most of the details are equally applicable to patients dying from other progressive disorders.

In compiling *Introducing Palliative Care*, I am acutely aware that the insights and information contained within it stem from many different people and sources, often long forgotten. One is reminded of the old saying that 'There is nothing new under the sun'. To my many anonymous teachers from the past, I express my gratitude. However, in the pages on communication and breaking bad news, the perceptive reader may well see the shadows of Ivan Lichter, Peter Maguire, and possibly others. By virtue of the shared authorship of *Symptom Management in Advanced Cancer* (third edition), I owe Andrew Wilcock a particular debt of gratitude. I am grateful to Julie Stokes and Winston's Wish for permission to include the *Charter for Bereaved Children* (Box 2.D), and to the following for permission to include various figures: Margaret Stroebe and Henk Schut (Figure 2.2), SIMS Graseby Limited (Figure 3.11) and the *British Medical Journal* (Figure 4.3).

The help of past and present colleagues is also acknowledged, particularly Jennifer Barraclough, David Cook, Val Hunkin, Karen Jenns, Suresh Kumar, Aslög Malmberg, Mary Miller, Michael Minton, MR Rajagopal, Fiona Randall, Ajitha Kumari, Victoria Slater, Rosalyn Staveley, Averil Stedeford and Sanjeev Vasudevan. Ann Couldrick, Marilyn Relf and Christine Pentland are named in the text as the principle contributors of the sections on bereavement. Thanks are also due to my secretary, Karen Allen, for preparing the typescript and to Susan Brown, copy editor, for her painstaking attention to detail.

Robert Twycross
October 2002

Drug names

Introducing Palliative Care uses recommended International Non-proprietary Names (rINNs). For about 150 drugs, the rINN differs from the British Approved Name (BAN). Following a European Union Directive, the use of BANs is being phased out and all drugs marketed in the UK will eventually be known by their rINNs. For drugs where there is a high risk of confusion, there will be a transition period during which both the BAN and the rINN must be used (Table 1). In the case of adrenaline (BAN), an exception has been made; in the UK, it will continue to have priority over epinephrine (rINN), i.e. will be prescribed as *adrenaline (epinephrine)*.

Table 1 Drugs relevant to palliative care for which both rINN and BAN must be used in the UK

rINN	*BAN*
Alimemazine	Trimeprazine
Bendroflumethiazide	Bendrofluazide
Calcitonin (salmon)	Salcatonin
Chlorphenamine	Chlorpheniramine
Epinephrine	*Adrenaline*
Dicycloverine	Dicyclomine
Dosulepin	Dothiepin
Furosemide	Frusemide
Levomepromazine	Methotrimeprazine
Lidocaine	Lignocaine
Mitoxantrone	Mitozantrone
Norepinephrine	*Noradrenaline*
Procaine benzylpenicillin	Procaine penicillin
Tetracaine	Amethocaine
Trihexyphenidyl	Benzhexol

For many drugs, the change is slight (e.g. danthron → dantron) but for others the rINN is very different (e.g. methotrimeprazine → levomepromazine). Certain general rules apply:

- 'ph' becomes 'f' (e.g. cephradine → cefradine)
- 'th' becomes 't' (e.g. indomethacin → indometacin)
- 'y' becomes 'i' (e.g. napsylate → napsilate).

However, there are many exceptions. Other affected drugs relevant to palliative care are listed in Table 2.

Table 2   Other drugs relevant to palliative care affected by European Union Directive

rINN	BAN
Amobarbital	Amylobarbitone
Amoxicillin	Amoxycillin
Beclometasone	Beclomethasone
Benorilate	Benorylate
Benzathine benzylpenicillin	Benzathine penicillin
Benzatropine	Benztropine
Cefalexin (etc.)	Cephalexin (etc.)
Ciclosporin	Cyclosporin
Clomethiazole	Chlormethiazole
Colestyramine	Cholestyramine
Dantron	Danthron
Dexamfetamine	Dexamphetamine
Dienestrol	Dienoestrol
Diethylstilbestrol	Stilboestrol
Dimeticone	Dimethicone
Estradiol	Oestradiol
Guaifenesin	Guaiphenesin
Indometacin	Indomethacin

continued

Table 2 *Continued*

rINN	BAN
Levothyroxine	Thyroxine
Methenamine hippurate	Hexamine hippurate
Oxetacaine	Oxethazine
Phenobarbital	Phenobarbitone
Retinol	Vitamin A
Sodium cromoglicate	Sodium cromoglycate
Sulfasalazine	Sulphasalazine
Sulfathiazole	Sulphathiazole

Outside Europe it is important to note several differences between rINNs and USANs, i.e. names used in the USA (Table 3). Note also that:

- diamorphine (available only in the UK) = di-acetylmorphine = heroin
- liquid paraffin = mineral oil.

Table 3 Important differences between rINNs and USANs

rINN	USAN
Dimeticone[a]	Simethicone
Dextropropoxyphene	Propoxyphene
Hyoscine hydrobromide	Scopolamine hydrobromide
Glycopyrronium	Glycopyrrolate
Paracetamol	Acetaminophen
Pethidine	Meperidine

a.   in some countries, dimeticone is called (di)methylpolysiloxane.

List of abbreviations

General

BNF	British National Formulary
BP	British Pharmacopoeia
MCA	Medicines Control Agency (UK)
rINN	recommended International Non-proprietary Name
UK	United Kingdom
USA	United States of America
USP	United States Pharmacopoeia
WHO	World Health Organization

Medical

CNS	central nervous system
COPD	chronic obstructive pulmonary disease
COX	cyclo-oxygenase; alternative, prostaglandin synthase
CSF	cerebrospinal fluid
CT	computed tomography
H_1, H_2	histamine type 1, type 2 (receptors)
INR	international normalised ratio
MAOI(s)	mono-amine oxidase inhibitor(s)
MRI	magnetic resonance imaging
NMDA	N-methyl D-aspartate
NSAID(s)	non-steroidal anti-inflammatory drug(s)
PCA	patient-controlled analgesia
PG(s)	prostaglandin(s)
PPI(s)	proton pump inhibitor(s)
SSRI(s)	selective serotonin re-uptake inhibitor(s)
TENS	transcutaneous electrical nerve stimulation

Drug administration

a.c.	ante cibum (before food)
amp	ampoule containing a single dose (cp. vial)
b.d.	bis die (twice daily); alternative, b.i.d.

CD	preparation subject to prescription requirements under The Misuse of Drugs Act (UK); for regulations see BNF
CIVI	continuous intravenous infusion
CSCI	continuous subcutaneous infusion
e/c	enteric-coated
ED	epidural
IM	intramuscular
IT	intrathecal
IV	intravenous
IVI	intravenous infusion
m/r	modified release; alternatives, slow release, controlled release
o.d.	omni die (daily, once a day)
o.m.	omni mane (in the morning)
o.n.	omni nocte (at bedtime)
OTC	over-the-counter (can be obtained without a prescription)
p.c.	post cibum (after food)
PO	per os, by mouth
POM	prescription only medicine
PR	per rectum
p.r.n.	pro re nata (as needed, when required)
PV	per vaginum
q.d.s.	quater die sumendus (four times a day); alternative, q.i.d.
q4h	quarta quaque hora (every 4 hours)
SC	subcutaneous
SL	sublingual
stat	immediately
t.d.s.	ter die sumendus (three times a day); alternative, t.i.d.
vial	sterile container with a rubber bung containing either a single or multiple doses (cp. amp)

Units

cm	centimetre(s)
cps	cycles per sec
dl	decilitre(s)
g	gram(s)
Gy	Gray(s), a measure of radiation
h	hour(s)
Hg	mercury
kg	kilogram(s)
L	litre(s)
mg	milligram(s)
ml	millilitre(s)

mm	millimetre(s)
mmol	millimole(s)
min	minute(s)
mosmol	milli-osmole(s)
nm	nanometre(s)
nmol	nanomole(s)
sec	second(s)

PART ONE

General topics

Fatal statistics · Palliative care · Quality of life
Specialist palliative care services · Dying at home
Ethical considerations · Appropriate treatment
Euthanasia · Hope

Fatal statistics

In recent years, specialist palliative care services have been established in an increasing number of countries, mainly in response to the needs of patients with incurable cancer. The incidence of cancer has increased considerably over the last 50 years because of tobacco smoking and greater life-expectancy (cancer is partly a disease of old age). At present:

- 1/3 of the population in the UK and the West develops cancer
- 1/4 of the population in the UK and the West dies of cancer.

Despite these gloomy figures, it is important to have a balanced view of cancer:

- the 5-year survival rate for all cancers has improved from 10% in 1960 to >50% in 2000[1]
- some cancers are completely cured, possibly as many as 1/3
- although 'spread to the liver' is widely thought to herald the beginning of the end, 16% of patients with colorectal cancer and a solitary liver metastasis at the time of diagnosis were alive 5 years later.[2]

Further, in one group of women with breast cancer, it was found that a fighting spirit or denial were associated with a better prognosis, and fatalism or helplessness and hopelessness with a worse prognosis.[3] However, other studies have not shown an association between attitude or mood and survival.[4]

The principles of palliative care are generally applicable to the care of patients with any type of life-threatening progressive disease. Indeed, in some countries, patients with acquired immune deficiency syndrome (AIDS) are major users of palliative care services.

Palliative care

Palliative care is the active total care of patients with life-limiting disease, and their families, by a multiprofessional team, when the disease is no longer responsive to curative or life-prolonging treatments. Hospice care is often used as a synonym for palliative care. However, in some countries, hospice care denotes community-based palliative care.

'Palliative' is derived from the Latin word *pallium*, a cloak. In palliative care, symptoms are 'cloaked' with treatments whose primary aim is to promote comfort. However, palliative care extends far beyond physical symptom relief; it seeks to integrate physical, psychological, social and spiritual aspects of care so that patients may come to terms with their impending death as fully and constructively as they can (Figure 1.1).[5] Its essence is poignantly reflected in a sentence from the Qur'an:

'May you be wrapped in tenderness, you my brother, as if in a cloak.'

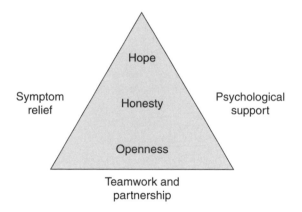

Figure 1.1   The three essential components of palliative care, bound together by the 'cement' of skilled communication.

'Supportive care' is sometimes used as an alternative to palliative care. The term was originally used to describe measures to combat the adverse effects of cancer treatment, such as anaemia, thrombocytopenia and neutropenic septicaemia. It is now used more widely to include rehabilitation and psychosocial support.[6] Thus, supportive care now embraces the same general domains as palliative care. However, for health professionals, policy makers and the general public, palliative care is synonymous with end-of-life care, whereas supportive care clearly has much wider application (Figure 1.2). Palliative care also extends, if necessary, to support in bereavement.

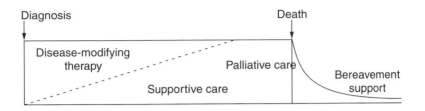

Figure 1.2 The relationship between disease-modifying therapy, supportive care and palliative care.

Palliative care is:

- patient-centred rather than disease-focused
- death accepting but also life-enhancing
- a partnership between the patient and the carers
- concerned with healing rather than curing.

Palliative care neither intentionally hastens nor intentionally postpones death.

Healing is about right relationships with self, others, environment and God: 'You can't die cured but you can die healed'.[7] To die healed means being able to say or convey:

'I love you,
Forgive me,
I forgive you,
Thank you,
Good-bye.'[8]

Palliative care is often said to be 'low tech and high touch'. It seeks to ensure that compassion and science are both governing forces in patient care. Accordingly, 'high tech' investigations and treatments are used only when their benefits clearly outweigh any potential burdens.

Rehabilitation

'Add life to their days, not days to their life.'

Palliative care is about quality of life (*see* p.5) and includes rehabilitation. It seeks to help patients achieve and maintain their maximum potential physically, psychologically, socially and spiritually, however limited these have become as a result of disease progression.

Teamwork

'Together Everyone Achieves More.'

Palliative care is best administered by a group of people working as a team. The team is collectively concerned with the total wellbeing of the patient and family. In practice, some or all of the following will be involved:

- doctor(s) and nurses (the essential core clinical team)
- physiotherapist, occupational therapist, other specific therapists
- social worker, chaplain/priest/rabbi, other advisers
- volunteers.

Because there is an overlap of roles, co-ordination is an important part of teamwork. Conflict inevitably erupts from time to time in a team of highly motivated, skilled professionals. One of the challenges of teamwork is how to handle conflict constructively and creatively. Volunteers are an integral part of most palliative care services, providing 'added value' as a result of their own life experiences and skills. They also form an important link with the wider community.

Partnership

The basis of palliative care is partnership between the caring team and the patient and family. Consultations should be seen as a meeting of experts: patients are the experts about how they feel and about the subjective impact of the illness and health professionals are the experts in diagnosis and management options. Partnership emphasises equality rather than hierarchy, and requires mutual respect (Box 1.A).

Box 1.A   Partnership with the patient

Be courteous and polite	Explain
Be honest	Agree priorities and goals
Don't be condescending	Discuss treatment options
Listen	Accept treatment refusal

'Care begins when difference is recognised. I reserve the name "caregivers" for the people who are willing to listen to ill persons and to respond to their individual experiences. Caring has nothing to do with categories. When the caregiver communicates to the ill person that she cares about the patient's uniqueness, she makes the person's life meaningful.'[9]

Quality of life

'Quality of life is what a person says it is.'

Quality of life relates to an individual's subjective satisfaction with life, and is influenced by all aspects of personhood: physical, psychological, social and spiritual. However, quality of life scores tend to be flawed because they measure only selected aspects and not global subjective satisfaction.[10,11]

In essence, there is good quality of life when the aspirations of an individual are matched and fulfilled by present experience. There is poor quality of life when there is a wide divergence between aspirations and present experience.[12] To improve quality of life, it is necessary to narrow the gap between aspirations and what is possible (Figure 1.3). Palliative care aims to do this.

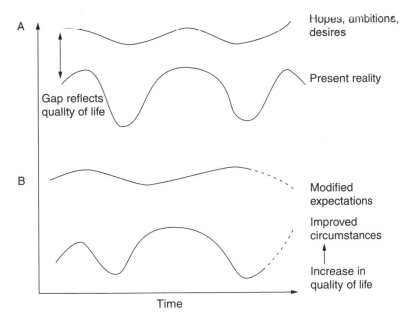

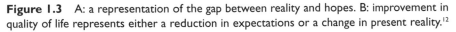

Figure 1.3 A: a representation of the gap between reality and hopes. B: improvement in quality of life represents either a reduction in expectations or a change in present reality.[12]

Thus, a tetraplegic ex-gymnastics instructor is able to say, 'The quality of life is excellent, though to see me you wouldn't believe it. I've come to terms with my loss and discovered the powers of my mind'. And a 30-year-old man dying of disseminated osteosarcoma complicated by paraplegia comments, 'The last year of my life has been the best'.

Specialist palliative care services

Although the emphasis is on home care, most palliative care centres in the UK offer a range of services, including:

- specialist home care nurses
- medical consultations
    at home with the general practitioner
    in other wards and hospitals
- outpatient clinics
- day care
- inpatient care
- bereavement support
- education (generally)
- research (sometimes).

Most inpatient services in the UK are provided by independent palliative care units (hospices), with a variable amount of funding from the NHS. The deficit, anything from 30–70% of the total cost, is made up from donations, legacies and active fundraising.

Clinical services are directed by a medical director/consultant physician and a matron/senior nurse. Typically in the UK, 90–95% of patients have cancer. However, in some countries, non-cancer patients account for up to 30%.

Home care

Specialist home care nurses (generally called Macmillan nurses in the UK) liaise with the primary healthcare team and offer advice on treatment and care. Because they provide support for the whole family, more patients are able to remain at home for longer or until death.

Day care

A palliative care day centre typically receives 10–15 patients a day. Patients are driven to and from the centre by volunteers. Patients attend for social support and to give the family a weekly respite. Medical and nursing care are also available. Basic services include bathing, hairdressing, manicure, chiropody and massage. Music therapy, art therapy and several other complementary therapies may also be available. The day centre enables many patients to remain longer at home. Those attending a day centre generally experience considerable improvement in morale, and find new meaning in life with restored hope as they benefit from the camaraderie, are given fresh opportunities for creative expression, and enjoy cultural activities.

Inpatient care

Patients are admitted for symptom management, for family relief (respite) or to die. About 1/2 of all admissions end with the patient returning home or to relatives. A high nurse-to-patient ratio is maintained because the physical and psychological needs of the patients are often considerable. Rehabilitation is facilitated by an occupational therapist and a physiotherapist. Inpatients are encouraged to make use of the facilities of the day centre. The median length of stay is typically 8–10 days.

Bereavement support

The primary healthcare team may well undertake this. However, support is often provided to 'high risk' survivors by trained volunteers under the supervision of a social worker or trained counsellor/psychologist. Each volunteer supports a limited number of bereaved relatives and other key carers. Support may also be given by the specialist home care nurses.

Education and research

Education is an important aspect of the work of a palliative care service. Various courses give opportunity for other health professionals to learn how to care better for patients with end-stage disease. Research is important if the care of dying patients is to be improved further. However, it is time-consuming and costly, and is undertaken successfully by relatively few centres.

Dying at home

If given the opportunity, most people would choose to die at home rather than in the alien environment of a hospital. With good support services, high quality care at home is often possible. It requires:

- a fit relative who can cope with serious illness
- nurses who can visit daily, or more often if necessary
- an attentive doctor
- a capability by the caring team to respond quickly to new problems
- a guarantee of rapid inpatient admission in the event of a major crisis.

Planning for the last days requires an understanding by the patient and the family of what might happen and of the sources for support which are available. It is vital for the psychological and physical wellbeing of the patient that, throughout the terminal phase, the doctor makes routine home visits and is available in the event of an emergency. It is important to indicate when the next routine visit will be:

> 'I'll call in again next Wednesday roundabout midday. If I can't, I'll telephone and let you know.'

Just emphasising that you are willing to visit at any time 'if there are problems' is *not* helpful. The patient and family do not feel supported; instead, they feel in limbo.

Most situations are manageable in the home and, although even the best laid plans may prove inadequate, families can often cope if they are able to talk at any time of the day or night with somebody who knows the patient. Families occasionally test out 24h availability and call for help at an unusual hour for some trivial reason. However, once they prove for themselves that somebody is really there, the service is rarely abused.

Particularly towards the end, the situation can change rapidly. Common problems, notably delirium (*see* p.155) and 'death rattle' (*see* p.129), should be discussed with the relatives so as to prepare them psychologically and practically. Although essential medication is likely to be given by continuous subcutaneous infusion (CSCI, *see* p.98), sometimes it may be necessary to discuss the practicality of rectal administration. A supply of drugs in suppository or injectable form should be kept in the home in case of an emergency such as a seizure or, in patients with head and neck cancer, massive haemorrhage.[13]

Despite initially expressing a wish to be cared for at home, many patients and families change their minds as the disease progresses. In a group of patients receiving specialist palliative care at home, preference for home care fell over time to about 50%.[14] Ultimately, less than 1/3 died at home; about the same proportion were admitted 1–3 days before death, and the rest for longer periods.

A person living alone or with an unfit relative generally needs to be admitted at some point. A prolonged terminal illness is also associated with eventual inpatient admission.[14]

Ethical considerations

The ethics of palliative care are those of medicine in general. Doctors have a dual responsibility to preserve life and to relieve suffering. At the end of life, as preserving life becomes increasingly impossible, relief of suffering is of even greater importance. Even so, even in palliative care, the intention is always to provide comfort and not to hasten death.

Four cardinal principles

- respect for patient autonomy (patient choice)
- beneficence (do good)
- non-maleficence (minimise harm)
- justice (fair use of available resources).[15]

The four cardinal principles need to be applied against a background of:

- respect for life
- acceptance of the ultimate inevitability of death.

In practice, there are three dichotomies which need to be applied in a balanced manner. Thus:

- the potential benefits of treatment must be balanced against the potential risks and burdens
- striving to preserve life but, when the burdens of life-sustaining treatments outweigh the potential benefits, withdrawing or withholding such treatments and providing comfort in dying
- individual needs are balanced against those of society.

Respect for patient autonomy

Doctors often act as if patients have an obligation to accept recommended treatment. However, legally a person is not obliged to accept medical treatment, even if refusal may result in an earlier death. Doctors have an obligation, therefore, to discuss treatment options and their implications with patients.

Without consent, a doctor risks being found liable in battery. In the UK, if a patient lacks capacity to give or withhold consent, a doctor's legal obligation is to treat in what he perceives as the patient's best interests. Severe depression, delirium (acute confusional state) or dementia are common causes of lack of capacity to give consent. A doctor, in common with any citizen, can restrain even a competent person in an emergency to prevent, for example, a crime or damage to other people.

Principle of double effect

'A single act having two possible foreseen effects, one good and one harmful, is not always morally prohibited if the harmful effect is not intended.'[16–19]

The principle of double effect is a universal principle without which the practice of medicine would be impossible. It follows inevitably from the fact that all treatment has an inherent risk. However, most discussions of the principle of double effect focus on the use of morphine or similar drugs to relieve pain in terminally ill patients. This gives the false impression that the use of morphine in this circumstance is a high risk strategy. When correctly used, morphine (and other strong opioids) are very safe drugs, safer than non-steroidal anti-inflammatory drugs, which are widely prescribed with impunity.[20] The use of both classes of analgesic is justified on the basis that the benefits of pain relief far outweigh the risk of serious undesirable effects. Indeed, clinical experience suggests that those whose pain is relieved live longer than would have been the case if they had continued to be exhausted and demoralised by severe unremitting pain.

The situation in the UK is encapsulated in a classic legal judgement:

> 'A doctor who is aiding the sick and the dying does not have to calculate in minutes or even in hours, and perhaps not in days or weeks, the effect upon a patient's life of the medicines which he administers or else be in peril of a charge of murder. If the first purpose of medicine, the restoration of health, can no longer be achieved, there is still much for a doctor to do, and he is entitled to do all that is proper and necessary to relieve pain and suffering, even if the measures he takes may incidentally shorten life.'[21]

Similar sentiments have been expressed in other countries, and reflect a broad international consensus.

However, the intended aim of treatment must be the relief of suffering and not the patient's death. Although a greater risk is acceptable in more extreme circumstances, it remains axiomatic that effective measures which carry less risk to life should normally be used. Thus, in an extreme situation, although it may occasionally be necessary and acceptable to render a patient unconscious, it remains unacceptable and unnecessary to cause death deliberately (euthanasia). Indeed, palliative care and euthanasia are essentially mutually exclusive philosophies.

Appropriate treatment

'Treatment that does not provide net benefit to the patient may, ethically and legally, be withheld or withdrawn and the goal of medicine should shift to the palliation of symptoms.'[22]

Doctors must keep in mind the fundamental fact that all patients must die eventually. Part of the skill of medicine, therefore, is to decide when to allow death to occur without further impediment. A doctor is not obliged legally or ethically to preserve life 'at all costs'. Priorities change when a patient is clearly dying. There is no obligation to employ treatments if their use can best be described as prolonging the process of dying.[23,24] A doctor has neither a duty nor the right to prescribe a lingering death. In palliative care, the primary aim of treatment is not to prolong life but to make the life which remains as comfortable and as meaningful as possible.

However, it is not a question of to treat or not to treat but what is the most appropriate treatment given the patient's biological prospects and his personal and social circumstances? Appropriate treatment for an acutely ill patient may be inappropriate in the dying (Figures 1.4 and 1.5). Nasogastric tubes, IV infusions, antibiotics, cardiac resuscitation, and artificial respiration are all primarily support measures for use in acute or acute-on-chronic illnesses to assist a patient through the initial crisis towards recovery of health. The use of these measures in patients who are irreversibly close to death is generally inappropriate (and therefore bad practice) because the burdens of such treatments exceed their potential benefits.

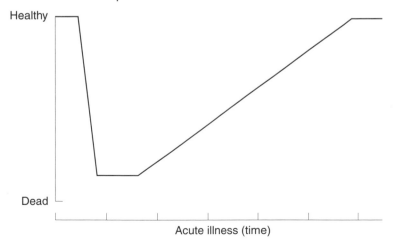

Figure 1.4   A graphical representation of acute illness. Biological prospects are generally good. Acute resuscitative measures are important and enable the patient to survive the initial crisis. Recovery is aided by the natural forces of healing; rehabilitation is completed by the patient on his own, without continued medical support.

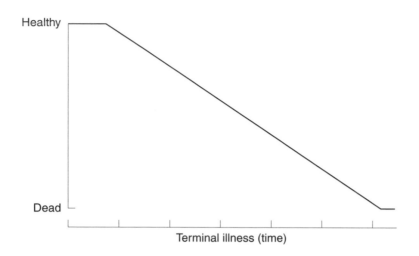

Figure 1.5   A graphical representation of terminal illness. Biological prospects progressively worsen. Acute and terminal illnesses are therefore distinct pathophysiological entities. Therapeutic interventions which can best be described as prolonging the distress of dying are futile and inappropriate.

Therapeutic recommendations are based on a consideration of the possible advantages (benefits) and disadvantages (risks and burdens) which might accrue for the patient. A doctor is not a technician and, in practice, there are generally several courses of action that might legitimately be adopted. Arguments in favour of a certain treatment revolve around the question of the anticipated effectiveness of intervention. Linked with this are considerations of the consequences and implications for the patient, the family and society as a whole. In other words, the doctor seeks, on the basis of the biological and social facts at his disposal, to offer the patient the most appropriate form of care. Remember, because death is inevitable for everybody, doctors ultimately have no choice but to 'let nature take its course'.

Medical care is a continuum, ranging from complete cure at one end to symptom relief at the other. Many types of treatment span the entire spectrum, notably radiotherapy and, to a lesser extent, chemotherapy and surgery. The therapeutic aim must be kept clearly in mind when employing any form of treatment. In deciding what is appropriate, the key points to bear in mind are:

- the patient's biological prospects
- the therapeutic aim and benefits of each treatment
- the undesirable effects of treatment
- the need not to prescribe a lingering death.

Although the possibility of unexpected improvement or recovery should not be totally ignored, there are many occasions when it is appropriate to 'give death a chance'. As death draws near, interest in hydration and nutrition often becomes minimal, and it is inappropriate to force someone to accept food and fluid. The patient's disinterest or positive disinclination is part of the process of letting go.

Euthanasia

Euthanasia literally means 'good death', death without suffering. However, in common parlance the word is used as a synonym for 'mercy killing'. Useful definitions include:

> 'A deliberate intervention undertaken with the express intention of ending a life to relieve intractable suffering.'[25]

> 'The compassion-motivated, deliberate, rapid and painless termination of the life of someone afflicted with an incurable and progressive disease. If performed at the dying person's request or with that person's consent, euthanasia is voluntary; otherwise it is non-voluntary.'[26]

Euthanasia is *not*:

- allowing nature to take its course
- stopping biologically futile treatment
- stopping treatment when the burdens outweigh the benefits
- using morphine and other drugs to relieve pain
- using sedatives to relieve intractable mental suffering in a dying patient.

The term passive euthanasia should not be used to describe 'letting nature take its course'. Withholding or withdrawing life-sustaining treatment when it is biologically futile or disproportionately burdensome is not euthanasia because it is not deliberate death acceleration; rather it is ceasing to prolong the patient's dying. The use of the term in this circumstance derives from a failure to distinguish between the aims of acute medicine and palliative care. Priorities change when a patient is expected to die within weeks or months; the primary aim is no longer prolonging life but achieving and maintaining comfort.

The term indirect euthanasia has been used to describe the administration of analgesics to patients with terminal cancer. This too is incorrect; giving a drug to lessen pain cannot be equated with giving a lethal overdose deliberately to end life.

The euthanasia debate

The debate about euthanasia within a plural society is generally conducted along pragmatic, utilitarian and consequentialist lines because to argue from mutually exclusive philosophical positions can never lead to the consensus which every society must strive for.

'We treat animals better than we do humans' and 'If he were an animal, he'd be put down' are comments which recur too often for comfort. Although on one level such comments can be easily countered, these statements reflect a depth of compassion and anguish which can easily be lost or ignored in a detached discussion of philosophical and ethical principles.

The fundamental argument in favour of euthanasia is a person's right to self-determination. The fundamental counter-argument is that autonomy does not extend to a right to medically-assisted suicide/euthanasia. These two viewpoints ('man as master' vs 'man as steward') are not reconcilable. Discussion concerning euthanasia generally assumes that death means oblivion. However, although many people believe otherwise, to make 'eternal destiny' the crucial argument in the case against euthanasia is generally unproductive.

Those in favour of euthanasia often stress that there is a level of existence where most, if not all, people would wish not to be kept alive. If conscious, they might actively ask for assistance to die, emphasising that life no longer has meaning or purpose for them. Patients in irreversible coma (more than 6 months?) would be one category and persistent vegetative state another; possibly, also advanced motor neurone disease (amyotrophic lateral sclerosis) or when cancer erodes the face and replaces familiar features with a malodorous ulcerating fungating mass, or when a similar process affects the perineum and results in distressing and humiliating double incontinence. These are powerful images and must be acknowledged by those who oppose euthanasia. Palliative care cannot 'sanitate' all forms of dying. Indeed, a doctor who:

- has never been tempted to kill a patient probably has had limited clinical experience or is not able to empathise with those who suffer
- leaves a patient to suffer intolerably is morally more reprehensible than the doctor who opts for euthanasia.

Requests for euthanasia

Persistent requests for euthanasia are uncommon.[27] Further, most of those who demand help to die are asking for help to live. It is critically important to hear the cry for life underlying the patient's 'lament'.[28] It is necessary, therefore, to identify the reasons for the demand and to respond accordingly.[27] Reasons vary but include:

- unrelieved severe pain or other physical distress, e.g. breathlessness or nausea and vomiting
- fear of future intolerable pain or other physical distress, e.g. suffocating or choking
- fear of a long slow deterioration over many months
- fear of being kept alive with machines and tubes at a time when quality of life would be unacceptably low, or when in coma
- a short-term adjustment disorder, i.e. temporary despair on discovering one has a fatal disease with limited life expectancy
- demoralisation (hopelessness, helplessness, 'no point in struggling on')
- depression (meaning a depressive illness, not just sadness or demoralisation)
- feeling a burden on one's family, friends, or society generally
- feeling unwanted by family, friends, or people generally
- being dependent on others and a feeling of no longer being in control
- a fixed feeling of hopelessness which cannot be explained in terms of any of the above, and which probably stems from a view of life which has no concept of personal survival beyond death.

With the exception of the last two, it is normally possible to improve the situation sufficiently for the person to change their mind.

The slippery slope

The 'slippery slope' is a term commonly used to refer to the danger of voluntary euthanasia for terminally ill patients leading to non-voluntary euthanasia and/or extending to patients who are not terminally ill. Despite strict guidelines, the experience in the Netherlands (where euthanasia and physician-assisted suicide are not criminal offences) appears to support this fear.[29,30]

A pragmatic approach

Because of opposition to euthanasia and physician-assisted suicide by the professionals involved, specialist palliative care is effectively 'a euthanasia-free zone'.[31] This fact needs to be taken into account in any discussion about euthanasia. Partly intuitive, this anti-euthanasia stance is sustained by pragmatic reasons (Table 1.1), and was reflected in the conclusion of a Parliamentary Select Committee on Medical Ethics in the UK:

'[There is] not sufficient reason to weaken society's prohibition of intentional killing which is the cornerstone of law and of social relationships.

Individual cases cannot reasonably establish the foundation of a policy which would have such serious and widespread repercussions. The issue of euthanasia is one in which the interests of the individual cannot be separated from those of society as a whole.'[32]

Table 1.1   Pragmatic reasons for opposing euthanasia

Reason	Comment
Prognosis is often uncertain	Some patients live for years longer than originally anticipated
Patients frequently change their minds	Many patients have transient periods of despair
Many requests stem from inadequate symptom relief	Patients stop asking when their symptoms are relieved adequately
Requests relate to a sense of uselessness or feeling a burden	Good palliative care restores hope by giving the patient a sense of direction and of connectedness with other people
Persistent requests often reflect a depressive illness	Depression necessitates specific treatment
A 'euthanasia mentality' results in voluntary euthanasia extending to non-voluntary euthanasia	This has happened in the Netherlands[33]
Once permitted, euthanasia will not be restricted to the terminally ill	Some supporters of euthanasia urge a wider application[34,35]
If voluntary euthanasia was permitted, elderly and terminally ill patients would feel 'at risk'	Anecdotal evidence supports this contention[36]
Pressure on doctors from relatives to impose euthanasia on patients could be irresistible	Anecdotal evidence supports this contention[37]
Doctors who find it hard to cope with 'failure' will tend to impose euthanasia	Anecdotal evidence supports this contention[29,38]
Budgetary constraints are seen by some to be a compelling reason for legalising euthanasia	This view has been expressed by both doctors and economists[39]
The option of euthanasia will remove the incentive to improve standards of palliative care	

Further, as someone said:

'Patients tend to be sedated when the carers have reached the limit of their resources and are no longer able to stand the patient's problems without anxiety, impatience, guilt, anger or despair. Perhaps many of the desperate treatments in medicine can be justified by expediency, but history has an awkward habit of judging some as fashions, more helpful to the therapist than to the patient.'[38]

Hope

'Hope is an expectation greater than zero of achieving a goal.'

Hope needs an object. Setting realistic goals jointly with a patient is one way of restoring and maintaining hope. Sometimes, it is necessary to break down an ultimate (probably unrealistic) goal into a series of (more realistic) 'mini-goals'. Thus, if a patient says, 'I want to be cured' or a paraplegic says, 'I want to walk again', an initial reply could be:

'I hear what you're saying … that is your ultimate goal. But I think it will be more helpful if we agreed on a series of short-term goals. Reaching these would give all of us a sense of achievement. How does that seem to you?'

Setting goals is an integral part of caring for patients with an incurable disease, even if progressive. In one study, doctors and nurses in two palliative care units set significantly more goals than did their counterparts in a general hospital.[40]

Hope is also related to other aspects of life and relationships (Table 1.2). Communication of painful truth does not equal destruction of hope (*see* p.25). Hope of recovery is replaced by alternative hopes. In patients close to death, hope tends to become focused on:

● being rather than achieving
● relationship with others
● relationship with God or a higher being.

Table 1.2 Factors that influence hope in the terminally ill[41]

Decrease	Increase
Feeling devalued	Feeling valued
Abandonment and isolation 'conspiracy of silence' 'conspiracy of words' 'there's nothing more that I can do for you'	Meaningful relationship(s) reminiscence humour
Lack of direction/goals	Realistic goals
Unrelieved pain and discomfort	Pain and symptom relief

It is possible, therefore, for hope to increase when a person is close to death, provided care and comfort remain satisfactory.[41] When little else is left to hope for, it should still be realistic to hope for a peaceful death.

References

1 Casciato D and Lowitz B (2000) *Manual of Clinical Oncology* (4e). Lippincott, Williams & Wilkins, Philadelphia.
2 Wood C (1984) Natural history of liver metastases. In: C Van De Velde and P Sugarbaker (eds) *Liver Metastases*. Martinus Nijhoff, Dordrecht, pp 47–54.
3 Pettingale K *et al.* (1985) Mental attitudes to cancer: an additional prognostic factor. *Lancet.* **i:** 750.
4 Lewis C *et al.* (2002) *The Psychoimmunology of Cancer* (2e). Oxford University Press, Oxford.
5 WHO (2002) *National Cancer Control Programmes. Policies and managerial guidelines* (2e). World Health Organization, Geneva, p. 84.
6 Senn H-J and Glaus A (2002) Supportive care in cancer – 15 years thereafter. *Supportive Care in Cancer.* **10:** 8–12.
7 Frimmer D (2000) *Time Magazine.* **September.**
8 LePoivedin S. Unpublished material.
9 Frank A (1991) *At the Will of the Body: reflections on illness.* Houghton Mifflin, Boston.
10 Twycross RG (1987) Quality before quantity. A note of caution. *Palliative Medicine.* **1:** 65–72.
11 Cohen S and Mount B (1992) Quality of life in terminal illness: defining and measuring subjective well-being in the dying. *Journal of Palliative Care.* **8(3):** 40–45.
12 Calman KC (1984) Quality of life in cancer patients – an hypothesis. *Journal of Medical Ethics.* **10:** 124–127.
13 LeGrand S *et al.* (2001) Dying at home: emergency medications for terminal symptoms. *American Journal of Hospice and Palliative Care.* **18:** 421–423.
14 Hinton J (1994) Can home care maintain an acceptable quality of life for patients with terminal cancer and their relatives? *Palliative Medicine.* **8:** 183–196.
15 Gillon R (1994) Medical ethics: four principles plus attention to scope. *British Medical Journal.* **309:** 184–188.
16 Beauchamp T and Childress J (1994) *Principles of Biomedical Ethics.* Oxford University Press, New York, pp 206–211.

17 Dunphy K (1998) Sedation and the smoking gun: double effect on trial. *Progress in Palliative Care.* **6:** 209–212.

18 Thorns A (1998) A review of the doctrine of double effect. *European Journal of Palliative Care.* **5:** 117–120.

19 Randall F and Downie R (1999) *Palliative Care Ethics. A companion for all specialties.* Oxford University Press, Oxford, pp 119–121.

20 Tramer M *et al.* (2000) Quantitative estimation of rare adverse events which follow a biological progression: a new model applied to chronic NSAID use. *Pain.* **85:** 169–182.

21 Devlin P (1985) *Easing the Passing. The trial of Dr John Bodkin Adams.* The Bodley Head, London, pp 171–182.

22 BMA (1999) *Withholding or Withdrawing Life-Prolonging Medical Treatment. Guidance for decision making.* BMA, London.

23 Gillon R (1999) End-of-life decisions. *Journal of Medical Ethics.* **25:** 435–436.

24 London D (2000) Withdrawing and withholding life-prolonging medical treatment from adult patients. *Journal of the Royal College of Physicians of London.* **34:** 122–124.

25 House of Lords (1994) *Report of the Select Committee on Medical Ethics. HL Paper 21-I.* HMSO, London.

26 Roy D and Rapin C (1994) Regarding euthanasia. *European Journal of Palliative Care.* **1:** 57–59.

27 Zylicz Z and Janssens M (1998) Options in palliative care: dealing with those who want to die. *Bailliere's Clinical Anaesthesiology.* **12:** 121–131.

28 Scott J (1992) Lamentation and euthanasia. *Humane Medicine.* **8:** 116–121.

29 Twycross RG (1996) Euthanasia: going Dutch. *Journal of the Royal Society of Medicine.* **89:** 61–63.

30 Foley K and Hendin H (2002) *The Case Against Assisted Suicide. For the right to end-of-life care.* Johns Hopkins University Press, Baltimore.

31 Farsides B (1998) Palliative care – a euthanasia-free zone? *Journal of Medical Ethics.* **24:** 149–150.

32 Walton J (1994) *Medical Ethics: Select Committe Report.* (Hansard), May 9, House of Lords, London, pp 1344–1349.

33 Van der Maas P *et al.* (1991) Euthanasia and other medical decisions concerning the end of life. *Lancet.* **338:** 669–674.

34 Smoker B (1991) Remember the non terminally ill and disabled. *Voluntary Euthanasia Society Newsletter.* **September:** 10.

35 Spanjer M (1994) Mental suffering as justification for euthanasia in Netherlands. *Lancet.* **343:** 1630.

36 Fenigsen R (1988) A case against Dutch euthanasia. *Hastings Center Report.* **19 (suppl):** 22s–30s.

37 Ministry of Justice *et al.* (1991) Report of the committee to investigate medical practice concerning euthanasia. Medical decisions about the end of life. II. *Euthanasia Survey Report.* The Hague.

38 Main T (1957) The ailment. *British Journal of Medical Psychology.* **30:** 129–145.

39 Bliss M (1990) Resources, the family and voluntary euthanasia. *British Journal of General Practice.* **40:** 117–122.

40 Lunt B and Neale C (1987) A comparison of hospice and hospital: care goals set by staff. *Palliative Medicine.* **1:** 136–148.

41 Herth K (1990) Fostering hope in terminally ill people. *Journal of Advanced Nursing.* **15:** 1250–1259.

PART TWO

Psychosocial aspects of care

Communication · Breaking bad news
Strategies for coping with uncertainty
Psychological aspects of terminal illness
The withdrawn patient · The difficult patient
Care of the relatives · Spiritual care · Religious needs
Bereavement · Children and bereavement

Communication

> 'Communications, like tumours, may be benign or malignant. They may also be invasive, and the effects of bad communication with a patient may metastasise to the family. Truth is one of the most powerful therapeutic agents available to us, but we still need to develop a proper understanding of its clinical pharmacology and to recognise optimum timing and dosage in its use. Similarly, we need to understand the closely related metabolisms of hope and denial.'[1]

The aims of communication are to:

- reduce uncertainty
- enhance relationships
- give the patient and family a direction in which to move.

The basic message a patient wants to hear at a time of increasing uncertainty is:

'No matter what happens to you, we will not desert you' (acceptance).
'You may be dying, but you are still important to us' (affirmation).

Only part of this can be said in words:

'We can relieve your pain and can ease most other symptoms.'
'I will see you regularly.'
'One of us will always be available.'
'Let's work out how best we can help you and your family.'

A large part of the message is conveyed to the patient by non-verbal means. Non-verbal communication includes:

- facial expression
- eye contact
- posture, including whether sitting or standing
- pitch and pace of voice
- touch.

'Cancer is isolating, and the isolation can hurt far more than the treatment. Suddenly, you, the person with cancer, find yourself on one side of the wall, the sick side. Everyone else in your world is on the other side of that wall, the normal side.'[2]

Touch is an important means of re-establishing a sense of connectedness with other people and with the world in general. A hand on the patient's hand or arm may be all that is needed to reduce the sense of isolation, although cultural norms should be borne in mind. Reducing the sense of isolation through touch explains why massage (including aromatherapy and reflexology) has a definite place in palliative care.

Getting started

- make time for an unhurried conversation without interruption
- privacy is important
- introduce self by name and shake hands
- sit down to indicate you have time to listen
- make eye contact
- avoid medical jargon.

Asking the patient to set the agenda is particularly important when the patient has many symptoms, which is often the case. A formal systematic enquiry may well leave the doctor uncertain as to what to tackle first, and add to the patient's distress because of the failure to develop a clear plan. Useful ways of starting include:

'How can I help you?'
'What would you like to tell me about first?'
'Please tell me about your problems.'
'What do you hope will come out of this consultation?'

It may be helpful for a new patient to tell their story from the start of illness, even if this was several years ago. For example, 'We've not met before; it would help me if you could start right from the beginning'. This often throws up unresolved concerns or resentments from the past which may be crucial to present management and support.

Active listening

- nod from time to time to show that you are still paying attention
- if the patient stops in the middle of a sentence, repeat her last three words; this gives permission to continue, and the offer is generally accepted
- pick up on cues, e.g. 'It's like Granny's illness'. 'What do you mean "It's like Granny's illness"?'
- reflect questions back, e.g. 'What do you think the operation was for?'
- ask about feelings, e.g. 'How did/does that make you feel?'
- validate feelings, e.g. 'It's natural you should feel like that'
- watch body language and pick up on non-verbal cues
- summarise to check the accuracy of your understanding of the patient's problems
- if there is a long list of problems, ask the patient to prioritise them.

Eliciting feelings vs distancing

One of the main aims of a consultation is to elicit the patient's feelings and concerns. Some questions tend to restrict the amount of information shared by the patient. Thus:

- *leading* questions tend to produce the answer the questioner wants to hear, e.g. 'Are you feeling better today?'
- *closed* questions tend to produce the answer yes or no, e.g. 'Have you any pain?'.

In contrast, open (*how* and *what*) questions allow the patient to express feelings and concerns, e.g.:

'How are you feeling today?'
'How have you been coping since we last met?'
'What worries you most about your situation?'
'What causes you the most suffering?'

Without open questions, it is generally impossible to discover how the patient is really feeling, and to find out what their main concerns are.

It is also important to avoid behaviours which block the expression of negative feelings and fears, or which increase frustration and resentment. Such behaviours are called 'distancing', i.e. behaviours by which caregivers avoid becoming involved with a patient on a psychosocial level. Some approaches may be helpful on one occasion but unhelpful on another, for example, posing questions or giving advice. However, some behaviours should never be used:

- issuing orders
- making threats
- moralising/lecturing
- making criticisms.

Doctors and other healthcare professionals are generally not aware when they are distancing.[3] Common ways by which doctors and others distance themselves include:

- non-verbal messages
    always busy
    facial expression
    tone of voice
- categorising or labelling, e.g.
    'She's a breast cancer'
    'He's a difficult patient'
- paying selective attention to 'safe' physical aspects
    Patient 'I'm getting very worried about myself. I'm losing weight and the pain in my back has come back again'
    Doctor 'Tell me about the pain'
- never enquiring beyond the physical, i.e. never asking
    'How are you feeling today?'
    'How have you been coping?'
- using only closed questions
- premature normalisation, e.g. when a patient starts to cry, saying
    'Don't worry, everyone in your position feels upset' instead of,
    'I can see you're upset. Can you tell me exactly what's upsetting you?'
- premature or false re-assurance, e.g.
    'Don't worry. You leave it to me. Everything will be all right'
- using euphemisms to mislead (a 'conspiracy of words')
- 'jollying along'/expecting the patient to keep up a brave face, e.g.
    'Come on, the sun's shining; there's no need to look so glum!'
- concentrating on physical tasks

- inappropriate humour
- disappearing from the stressful situation.

Peoples ability to express thoughts and feelings, particularly negative ones, varies greatly. For some people, deep verbal communication is virtually impossible. However, they may obtain considerable benefit from non-verbal expression, e.g. through music or art therapy.

Breaking bad news

Bad news is information that drastically and unpleasantly alters a patient's view of her future. In practice, it is seldom a question of 'to tell or not to tell', but more a matter of 'when and how to tell'.

Breaking bad news generally causes distress to both the patient and the newsgiver. It is necessary to be prepared for a strong emotional reaction, e.g. tears, anger. Telling the patient and family together avoids difficulties and mistrust. It also gives the opportunity for mutual support.

The dictum 'never destroy hope' is sometimes used as a reason for not informing a patient of the seriousness of the situation. However, false optimism is a potent destroyer of hope. On the other hand, a total catharsis of all that is negative by the doctor, either to the patient or to the family, may irreversibly destroy hope and result in intractable anxiety and despair. It is necessary, therefore, to apply two parallel principles, namely:

- never lie to a patient
- avoid thoughtless candour.

Gradual communication of the truth within the context of continued support and encouragement almost always leads to enhanced hope (see p.17). The doctor–patient relationship is founded on trust. It is nurtured by honesty but poisoned by deceit.

The doctor's relationship with the patient should not be compromised by making unwise (and unethical) promises to the relatives about not informing the patient. It is necessary to check awareness, i.e. where the patient is at present in terms of knowledge and understanding, and to proceed according to her responses.

If a patient indicates directly or indirectly that she does not wish to regard her illness as fatal, it is wrong to force the truth on her. She is using denial as a coping strategy and, as such, it is vital to her present wellbeing. However, few patients adopt such a stance permanently.

Patients who want to know more about their condition often ask indirectly:

'And what's the next step, doctor?'
'How long do you reckon this will go on, doctor?'
'I'm not getting any better, am I?'

Sometimes it is necessary to use questions to find out if a patient wants more information:

'What things have been running through your mind as to the underlying cause of your symptoms?'
'This illness is dragging on. Do you ever find yourself looking on the black side of things?'

Alternatively, it may be helpful to ask the patient:

'Are you the sort of person who likes to know what's happening or do you prefer to leave it all to the doctors?'

If the patient indicates that they prefer to 'leave it to the doctor', this should be accepted as the present position. However, the patient should be advised that they are free to ask questions at any time should they wish to.

If the patient wants more information:

● give a 'warning shot' before stating the diagnosis, e.g. 'Tests indicate that we could be dealing with something serious'
● tailor the information to the patient's perceived needs, sometimes using a series of euphemisms, e.g. 'some abnormal cells', 'a kind of tumour', 'a bit cancerous', as a way of moving gently but definitely towards the explicit use of the word 'cancer'
● stop if the patient indicates that they have heard enough, e.g. 'Well, I'll leave all that in your hands, doctor'.

But remember that doctors generally underestimate what patients already know.

For most people, cancer is an emotive word. If a patient with incurable cancer asks directly, 'Have I got cancer?', first discover what they understand by 'cancer'. If it means an agonising death, it is important to explain that this will not be the case because treatments are now available to relieve pain and other symptoms should they develop.

After giving bad news, try to offer some good news; but not before finding out how the patient feels about the bad news. Good news might include:

● information about possible further anticancer treatment

- they still have a future despite the cancer being incurable
- there will still be good times ahead despite progressive illness
- there is much that can be done to relieve pain and other distressing symptoms.

Truth has a broad spectrum with gentleness at one end and harshness at the other. People prefer gentle truth. As far as possible, soften the initial impact of emotionally negative words:

Not	'You've got cancer.'	*But*	'Tests indicate that it is a form of cancer.'
Not	'You've got 3 months to live.'	*But*	'Time is probably limited.'

Use words with positive rather than negative overtones:

Not	'You've got weaker.'	*But*	'Energy, at the moment, is in short supply.'
Not	'Things are getting worse.'	*But*	'Things don't seem to be so good this week.'

Euphemisms are legitimate if used to express truth gently; they are wrong if used to deceive. Anger is a normal response to bad news and may be directed at the doctor. It is important not to become defensive. Instead, listen carefully to what is being expressed, clarify the causes and indicate that: 'Given what you're having to cope with, you've every right to be angry'. Judgements about the appropriateness of the focus of the anger are not helpful.

In summary

- location: get the physical surroundings right, e.g. privacy
- find out what the patient knows
- find out what the patient wants to know
- share information
    use open questions to facilitate the expression of the patient's concerns
    do not give false hope
    do not give more information than is wanted
    do not be afraid of silence
    check back to ensure that the message has been taken in
    make sure you are answering the question being asked
    have the confidence to say, 'I don't know'
    try to get the patient to come to their own conclusion

accept denial but do not collude with it, 'Perhaps we'd better just wait and see'

stress what medical science can offer, perhaps erring on the side of optimism

acknowledge the awfulness of uncertainty and explore the problems it creates (*see* below)

- allow the expression of strong emotions, e.g. tears, anger
- arrange to meet again to deal with any 'matters arising'.

Remember: not talking will not prevent the inevitable from happening. Be honest with yourself; recognise that when you say that you want to protect the patient, it generally means that you are trying to protect yourself.

Strategies for coping with uncertainty

Prognosis depends on many different factors, both physical and psychological. Although mean and median figures for survival may be available, these relate to 'Mr/Ms Average' and not to the patient sitting in front of you. When a patient asks about prognosis, try to avoid giving a specific length of time:

Patient 'How long have I got, doctor?'
Doctor 'I don't know ... nobody knows ... there are just too many factors to take into account, both physical and psychological ... I don't know'.

Many terminally ill patients die sooner than the doctor's estimate.[4] If given a specific time, some patients act as if the doctor's estimate is a divine prophecy. In consequence, they become increasingly fearful as the 'deadline' approaches and, indeed, may suffer some fatal cardiovascular or other catastrophe on the day of their predicted death.

Having established that nobody knows, it is important to:

- ask the patient what made them ask; this may unearth specific concerns which can then be discussed
- acknowledge that living with uncertainty is very difficult; 'That's hard isn't it ... having to live with the uncertainty?'
- discuss coping strategies
  a rolling horizon
  hope for the best but plan for the worst
  reaching anniversaries
  living one day at a time.

A rolling horizon

Here the anticipated survival is 4–6 months or more:

> 'Given how you are now, you should work on the basis that you'll be well enough to do what you want to do for the next 2–3 months. So go home and fill your diary out for this period of time, with the high expectation that you'll be able to fulfil your commitments. If in 4 weeks time, you're still as good as you are now, or better, then fill your diary out for another month, and so on'.

Hope for the best but plan for the worst

Here the anticipated survival is about 2–3 months:

> 'Given how things have been and are now, it is difficult to plan confidently for the future. What I suggest is that you adopt a "cross-eyed" approach: with one eye plan as if things are going to work out fairly well and, with the other, make alternative plans in case things don't work out so well … How does that seem to you?'.

Reaching anniversaries

Here the outlook seems very poor, but the patient is still hoping for some time. In this circumstance, it may help to identify anniversaries or special events which will occur in the next few months, and suggest to the patient that she should aim to reach them one by one.

Living one day at a time

Some people do this successfully for months, but it can lead to wasted time and opportunities because the patient sets no medium-term goals. However, in people who are within a few weeks of death, it is often a helpful strategy. An alternative, in less ill patients, is to suggest living 1–2 weeks at a time.

Beware the tendency of some patients to 'extremise':

> Doctor   'It could be 2–3 months or it could be 2–3 years.'
> Patient   (later to family) 'The doctor said I had only 2 months to live', or 'The doctor said I had at least 3 years'.

When pressed for more information, remember that with cancer:

- if deteriorating *month by month*, the prognosis is likely to be *months*
- if deteriorating *week by week*, the prognosis is likely to be *weeks*
- if deteriorating *day by day*, the prognosis is likely to be *days*.

But how long is *months, weeks, days*? With other end-stage diseases, it is even harder to prognosticate because of a patient's ability to pull back from yet another acute-on-chronic exacerbation or superadded infection.

Psychological aspects of terminal illness

Similar psychological responses occur with major losses of any kind, e.g. loss of a job, amputation, divorce, bereavement, as well as the anticipated loss of one's own life (Table 2.1). These responses do not necessarily occur in sequence. Several may occur together and some may not occur at all. Oscillations in the patient's feelings are common. In cancer patients, more marked responses are often seen:

- at or shortly after the time of diagnosis
- at the time of the first recurrence
- as death approaches.

Table 2.1   Psychological responses to loss[5]

Phase	Symptoms	Typical duration
Disruption	Disbelief Denial Shock/numbness Despair	Days → weeks
Dysphoria	Anxiety Insomnia Poor concentration Anger Guilt Activities disrupted Sadness Depression	Weeks → months
Adaptation	(as dysphoria diminishes) Implications confronted New goals established Hope refocused and restored Activities resumed	Months

Denial

'A psychological anaesthetic to an otherwise unbearable reality.'
'The psychological shock-absorber that allows us to suppress mentally what we cannot accept emotionally.'

Denial is a common defence mechanism. It signifies an ability to obliterate or minimise threatening reality by ignoring it. However, it may be associated with physiological and other non-verbal evidence of anxiety.

Most patients and relatives continue to make a fluctuating use of denial, reflecting a conflict between the wish to know the truth and the wish to avoid anxiety. Specific intervention may be needed if denial persists and interferes with:

- the acceptance of treatment
- planning for the future
- interpersonal relationships.

Anger

Anger may be an appropriate short-term reaction to the diagnosis of serious illness, but persistent anger is a problem. If anger is displaced or projected onto the family or staff, it tends to alienate those who want to give care. Anger can also interfere with the acceptance of limitations, and may stop a patient from making positive adjustments to physical disability. If anger is suppressed, the patient may become withdrawn, unco-operative or depressed.

Anxiety

Anxiety often relates to uncertainty and fear of the future, and the threat of separation from loved ones. Severe anxiety is accompanied by physical symptoms, such as palpitations, breathlessness, dry mouth, dysphagia, anorexia, nausea, diarrhoea, frequency of micturition, dizziness, sweating, tremor, headache, muscle tension, fatigue, weakness of the legs and chest pain. Many anxious patients sleep badly, have frightening dreams, or are reluctant to be left alone at night.

Depression

Recognising depression is important because patients often have a good response to antidepressant drugs. However, depression is often missed because symptoms overlap with appropriate grief about dying (sadness), with demoralisation (hopelessness, helplessness, 'no point in struggling on') and with the somatic symptoms of the cancer (anorexia, constipation, weight loss). Many patients also try to hide their negative feelings. Pointers to depression include:

- persistent low mood for >2 weeks, but possibly with diurnal variation
- loss of interest and inability to feel pleasure (anhedonia)
- feelings of guilt or unworthiness
- hopelessness/despair
- physical manifestations of anxiety, e.g. sweating, tremor, panic attacks
- suicidal attempts/persistent thoughts about suicide
- requests for euthanasia.

Paranoid states

Paranoid states may be caused by corticosteroids, a biochemical disturbance, cerebral metastases or psychological factors. For example, unable to accept that they are dying, patients may believe that there is a plot to kill them or that their deterioration is caused by the treatment.

Family problems

Cancer always changes family psychodynamics, either for better or worse. Within families, there is a conflict between the wish to confide and to receive emotional and practical support on the one hand and the wish to protect loved ones from distress on the other, particularly children or frail parents. A conspiracy of silence (collusion) is a source of tension. It blocks discussion of the future and preparation for parting. If it is not resolved, the bereaved often experience much regret.

Other problems

Cancer-related e.g. impact on sexual function, difficulty in accepting a colostomy, paraplegia or the effects of cerebral secondaries.

Treatment-related e.g. hair loss. Fear of death may make some patients want to go on with anticancer treatment even when undesirable effects are severe and the chance of improvement is minimal. Others may wish to opt for a shorter life with better quality when doctors are advocating more aggressive measures.

Concurrent e.g. a bereavement or a pre-existing psychiatric illness.

Management

Psychological problems are often missed by doctors and nurses. About 15% have an identifiable depressive illness.[6] Problems are also common among patients' relatives. Open questions, e.g. 'How are you feeling?' and 'How are you coping?' may facilitate the expression of much negative emotion. Useful questions which may reveal depression include:

'What has your mood been like lately?'
'Are you depressed?'
'Have you had a serious depression before? Are things like that now?'

Remember the adage: 'a trouble shared is a trouble halved'. This is particularly true in relation to worries, fears, and anger.

Some psychological problems can be prevented by:

● good staff–patient communication, giving information according to individual need (unfortunately, patients and families are not always given the information they are seeking, even when asked directly)
● good staff–patient relationships, with continuity of care
● allowing patients to have some control over the management of their illness.

There is no one right way of responding and adjusting to a poor prognosis. The doctor's task is to help the patient adjust in the best way possible, given that particular patient's family, cultural and spiritual background. Many people have a combination of inner resources and good support from the family and others which enable them to cope without prolonged and disabling distress.

Some patients benefit from specific relaxation therapy and, for others, an anxiolytic or an antidepressant is necessary. Specialist psychological interventions may be necessary for, *inter alia*, war veterans, holocaust survivors and those who have been abused or tortured.

The withdrawn patient

Some patients seem to be psychologically inaccessible. Although this may not be detrimental to the patient, there are times when the patient's facial expression and behaviour suggest considerable underlying psychological distress.

Causes

These fall into several categories (Box 2.A). Sometimes there may be several concurrent causal factors.

```
┌─────────────────────────────────────────────────────────────────┐
│ Box 2.A   Differential diagnosis of the withdrawn patient⁷       │
├─────────────────────────────────────────────────────────────────┤
```

Personality

Pathological
Brain tumour(s)
Cerebrovascular disease
Secondary mental disorders (see p.153)
Concurrent illness, e.g. hypothyroidism

Pharmacological
Oversedation
Tardive dyskinesia

Psychological

Anger	⎫	
Collusion	⎬	'no point in talking about my feelings'
Distrust	⎭	
Fear		'too painful'
Guilt	⎫	'too embarrassed'
Shame	⎭	

Psychiatric

| Depression | 'no point in talking about my feelings' |
| Paranoia | 'too dangerous' |

Management

Management depends on the cause. If a psychological cause seems likely, try to find a 'window' in the patient's protective shell in order to help them acknowledge the problem and to begin to move forward to a healthier/more comfortable frame of mind. Good communication skills are essential to achieve this:

- acknowledge your difficulty, 'We seem to be finding it difficult to get into conversation'
- offer the patient an invitation which they can accept or reject, e.g. 'Are you able to tell me why you find it difficult to talk to me about things?'

- if the patient then gives a clue as to the reason for the reticence, this should be gently but firmly followed up, e.g. 'Can you tell me exactly what's troubling you?'
- it is important to establish the frequency and intensity of any mood disturbance in case the patient is psychiatrically ill rather than just psychologically disturbed
- ask for specialist help if you feel you are getting nowhere.

The difficult patient

It is not possible to be equally positive towards all patients. Some patients we find difficult. It is important to remember that the problem is primarily *ours* and not the patient's, although it could be a joint problem. Thus, it is better to say, 'I find Mrs Brown difficult to look after' and not, 'Mrs Brown is difficult'.

Causes

There are many reasons why a patient may be difficult to care for (Box 2.B). The difficulties elicit feelings of impotence and inadequacy in us; we feel we have failed and that we have come to the end of our therapeutic resources.

Box 2.B   Reasons why patients can be difficult to care for

Patients or relatives perceived as
Unpleasant
Seductive
Ungrateful
Critical
Antagonistic
Demanding
Manipulative
Overdependent

Patient's behaviour
Withdrawn
Psychologically volatile, angry
Depressed

Patient's symptoms
Gross disfigurement
Malodour
Poor response to symptom
    management
Somatisation

Transference and countertransference

Management

- acknowledge your difficulty with the rest of the team
- explore possible reasons why the patient seems difficult.

Consider transference and countertransference reactions, i.e. negative feelings evoked by behaviour or personality traits in the patient because of your past experiences (transference), or your personality evoking negative feelings in the patient (countertransference). Both parties sense the negative 'vibes' and react to them.

Agree on a management plan with the rest of the team and record it in the notes, including short-term goals and time to be spent with the patient and family. Accept that some problems cannot be solved.

Care of the relatives

The care of the family is an integral part of the care of the dying. A contented family increases the likelihood of a contented patient. Relative–doctor communication generally needs to be initiated and maintained by the doctor. It is easy to neglect the family because they are reluctant to trouble the doctor 'because he's so busy'.

Telling the relatives

For the family and patient to be too far out of step in relation to knowledge about the diagnosis and the prognosis can create a barrier between them. A common initial reaction is, 'You won't tell him, will you, doctor?' or 'We'd prefer you not to tell him, doctor'. This should be seen as an initial shock reaction, stemming from the relative's own instinctive fear of death coupled with a desire to protect a loved one from hurt. It should not be used as an excuse for saying nothing to the patient.

If the family and patient are to be mutually supportive it is necessary to help the relatives move forward from this initial reaction to a position of greater openness and trust. The family cannot forbid the doctor from discussing diagnosis and prognosis with the patient. Indeed, given the ethic of medical confidentiality, it is clear that relatives can be told only with the implicit or explicit permission of the patient, and not the other way round.

In practice, there is much to be said for joint interviews at the time of diagnosis and later, i.e. patient, relative, doctor and nurse. This prevents collusion and a conspiracy of silence by which the patient is excluded from the process of information sharing. In addition, the presence of a nurse facilitates subsequent clarification of what the doctor said.

The doctor should also make an opportunity to see both the patient and the close family apart from each other. Further separate or joint interviews can then be arranged as necessary. As with the patient, it is generally unwise to tell the family initially the whole truth (as you perceive it); they also need time to adjust to the implications of the diagnosis.

Involvement in inpatient care

Admission to hospital or a palliative care unit may be seen as a defeat by the family. It helps if it is emphasised that it is remarkable that they have managed to cope for so long and now, with the need for 24h care, it is impossible to continue without a break. It should also be emphasised that the presence of relatives and close friends is regarded as important for the patient's continued wellbeing. If practical, unrestricted visits should be encouraged.

The relatives' separation anxiety may be reduced by encouraging them to continue to help in the care of the patient, e.g. by adjusting pillows, refilling a water jug, assisting at meals, helping with a blanket bath, Some relatives need to be taught how to visit, e.g. to behave as if they were at home and to sit and read a book or newspaper, knit, or watch the television together. They need to know that they don't have to keep up a tiring patter of conversation.

Overnight accommodation should be arranged when necessary, possibly using a divan in the patient's room, or guest accommodation if available.

Planning for discharge

A proportion of patients with terminal illness, particularly cancer, improve following admission as a result of pain and symptom management. They become physically independent and no longer need to be inpatients. Many relatives have fears about what will happen should the patient be discharged. A daytime visit or a weekend at home often does much to allay their fears, or confirms after all that discharge is impractical. A doctor (as well as other team members) should discuss matters with the relatives both before and after a trial period at home. Future plans can then be made on the basis of comments by both the family and the patient.

Patients are sometimes overprotected by their family. For example, even though still capable of driving, visiting the pub or betting shop, they are not allowed to do so. It is necessary in these cases to help the relatives to accept the patient's need (and right) to maintain the maximum possible degree of independence. An explanation that a sudden deterioration is unlikely will help to ease the family's apprehension. They also need guidance about who to call in an emergency, the general practitioner or the palliative care service.

Explanation of treatment

Terminally, the relatives should be warned that, if swallowing becomes difficult, it may be necessary to give medication by injection (or suppository) to prevent pain or other symptoms from recurring. If pneumonia develops, the doctor should explain that he plans to treat it symptomatically and not use antibiotics.

After the patient's death

Because bereavement has both a morbidity and a mortality, palliative care does not end when the patient dies. Many relatives have false feelings of guilt:

'If only I'd done this!'
'If he'd gone to the hospital sooner, maybe he wouldn't have died?'

Opportunity should be given for such feelings to be aired.

Spiritual care

'Spirituality is the valuing of the non-material aspects of life, and intimations of an enduring reality.'
'The sense of wonder – that is the sixth sense.'

Spirituality can be defined as *awareness of the transcendent*, the awareness of something beyond ordinary human knowledge or experience.[8]

Glimpses of spirituality at Sir Michael Sobell House[9]
In talking together about spirituality, a rich mixture of experiences, insights and feelings has emerged which defy simple definition. There is both meaning and mystery, a sense of interconnectedness and relationship alongside an awareness of our individuality.

We may connect with the spiritual through the beauty of the natural world, through our relationships with others, through religious practices, through painting or music, or through other forms of art.

continued

> But there is also a sense of awe and aloneness on this journey. We may have faith, and we may search and question. Our feelings may shift from courage and hope to fear, and back again. There may be joy, love, forgiveness, and truth, as well as pain and suffering. Through all, a dynamic energy takes us along our different paths. It is an area of experience where we may have more to learn from patients and relatives than we have to teach, more to receive than to give.

Spirituality is not limited to one discrete dimension of being human in the world but concerns the whole of life (Figure 2.1).

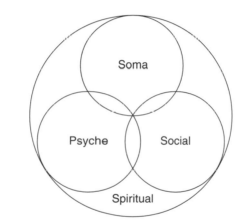

Figure 2.1   The 4S model of the human being; the spiritual dimension embraces and integrates the physical, psychological and social dimensions.

Spirituality engages the fundamental questions:

'What does it mean to be fully human in my particular circumstances?'
'What does it mean to be whole?'

Spirituality is thus concerned with:

- meaning and purpose in life
- interconnectedness and harmony with other people, planet Earth and the universe
- right relationship with God/Ultimate Reality.

For people facing death, such concerns tend to be brought into sharp focus.

Although often intermingled, spirituality and religion are not the same. It is possible to have either a secular spirituality or a religious spirituality.[10] A religion is a shared framework of theistic beliefs and rituals which give expression to spiritual concerns. It is also a social context in which spirituality is nurtured, the meaning of life is explored and identity formed.

For those nearing the end of life, there is commonly an increased or renewed need for:

- affirmation and acceptance
- forgiveness and reconciliation ('completion', see p.3)
- the discovery of meaning and direction.

Death is not the ultimate tragedy of life, depersonalisation is:

- dying in an alien and sterile area
- separation from the spiritual nourishment of fellow humans by a 'conspiracy of silence' (see p.32)
- helplessness, hopelessness and despair.

Whether apparent or not, most patients are in need of spiritual help and are seeking answers:[11]

> *Meaning of suffering and pain* 'Why do I have to suffer?' 'Why has this happened to me?'
> *Value systems* 'What value is there in money, material possessions, and social position?' 'What is valuable in my life?'
> *Quest after God* 'Is there a God?' 'Why does God allow me to suffer like this?'
> *The meaning of life* 'What is the meaning of life in a time of serious illness?' 'What's the point of it all?' 'What is my relationship with God?'
> *Guilt feelings* 'I've done many wrong things. How can they be put right? Can I be forgiven?'
> *Life after death* 'Is there life after death?' 'How can I believe in life after death?' 'What's it like?'

Few patients spontaneously discuss the spiritual aspects of life and death with their doctor but many do so with another team member, or with relatives and close friends. The following questions facilitate communication at this level:

> 'What or who do you find most supportive when life is difficult, like now?'
> 'What role does religion play in your life?'[12,13]

Patients are generally very perceptive and are unlikely to embarrass a doctor (or other carer) if they sense that communication at this level will cause discomfort. However, if a patient does and you feel uncomfortable, ask the patient if you may share what they have said with the chaplain or another team member.

A doctor's primary responsibility is to help maintain an environment which is supportive of the patient. This includes the relief of symptoms so that the patient is able to reflect on life and its meaning. However, it is important to recognise that some intractable symptoms reflect unexpressed spiritual distress, and that deliberate, specific enquiry may be indicated.

A note of caution: it is important not to think that you understand the spiritual pain a patient is suffering. Each of us has to find answers to the challenges of life which are personally satisfying. Thus, providing neat answers to a patient's questions is unlikely to be helpful. Sharing in not knowing may well be more comforting for the patient than being left feeling that other people have all the answers.

Further, respect for patients as individuals does not allow the imposition on them of one's own faith (or lack of it). Even so, many patients are comforted by the discovery that their doctor (or other carer) has a religious faith.

Some possible indicators of spiritual need, pain or dis-ease[14]

- sense of hopelessness, helplessness, meaninglessness (patients may become withdrawn and suicidal); 'I'd be better off dead than living like this', 'What's the point of going on like this?'
- intense suffering (includes loneliness, isolation, vulnerability); 'I can't endure this any more', 'If this is the best you can do, I'd rather be dead'
- remoteness of God, break with religious ties; 'I don't believe in God any more', 'I can't ask him for help'
- anger towards God, religion, clergy; 'Why? Why me?', 'What have I done to deserve this?'
- undue stoicism and desire to show others how to do it; 'I must not let God/ my church/my family down'
- a sense of guilt or shame (illness means punishment), bitter and unforgiving of self/others, 'I don't deserve to get better'
- vivid dreams/nightmares, e.g. about being trapped in a box or falling into a bottomless pit.

Any illness tends to concentrate the mind and raise questions of what is beyond death, e.g. letting go into what?

Religious needs

Broadly speaking, the impact of a person's religion is either *life-enhancing* or *life-escaping*.[15] These two types are represented in the adherents of all religions. Life-enhancing religion is generally supportive in the face of illness and death; life-escaping religion often is not, and may well increase fear and distress.

Further, those who accept a specific religious label are often not wholly orthodox in their beliefs. Thus, a Christian or a Muslim, for example, may not believe certain dogmas contained within the official statements of belief. In other words, a specific religious label does not necessarily mean a specific set of personal beliefs. As always, listen to the patient and don't make unwarranted assumptions.

In the UK, most hospitals, and probably all palliative care units, have a chapel. Many patients value its peace and quiet, 'I feel a lot better after sitting here in the chapel'. Several useful books are available which summarise the beliefs of the major world religions.[16,17] These can be consulted when necessary.

The following should be noted:

- *modesty,* most ethnic Asians, and Muslims of any ethnic background, would find it very distressing to be bathed by a nurse not of the same gender, many Asian women dislike undressing for physical examination
- *advanced directives/'do not resuscitate',* generally allowed but some sects within a faith tradition may forbid
- *medication,* some Buddhists and some Hindus may decline analgesics or sedatives
- *blood transfusions,* Jehovah's Witnesses (a Christian sect) are forbidden to receive blood transfusions
- *organ donation,* some restrictions for Jews
- *autopsy,* allowed for Jews and Muslims only if legally required; distasteful for Hindus
- *disposal of corpse,* burial within 24h for Jews and Muslims (no embalment); cremation for Sikhs and most Hindus; burial or cremation for Buddhists and Christians
- *belief in after-life,* resurrection in heaven, Christians, Jews and Muslims; rebirth for Buddhists;[18] re-incarnation for Hindus and Sikhs.

Dietary restrictions

Muslims and Sikhs do not drink alcohol, and may decline medicinal solutions if they contain alcohol. Some Buddhists and many Hindus and Sikhs are vegetarian. Most Hindus never eat beef (cows are sacred) and, for some, food should normally be prepared by a member of the same caste. Sikhs never eat meat that is halal, i.e. killed in the approved way for Muslims, and most do not eat beef. Jews and Muslims do not eat pork or shellfish. Orthodox Jews eat meat only if it has been killed by their own trained people (Kosher); some hospitals store deep-frozen Kosher meals.

Buddhism

Helping people is fundamental to the Buddhist ideal and the patient will always respect those (doctor, nurse, etc.) helping him. The family should be consulted whenever possible about specific wishes or needs. It may be possible to contact a local Buddhist monk when a Buddhist is dying.

A Buddhist may wish to maintain clarity of thought as long as possible while dying, and may decline medication if this is likely to induce drowsiness.[19] Anyone may prepare the body for burial/cremation. Black or white is the colour of mourning.

Christianity

A Christian priest or minister will normally have been visiting regularly, often sharing responsibilities with the hospital or palliative care chaplain. For some, readings from the Bible and prayer is preferred, but many appreciate receiving the relevant sacraments (rituals), e.g. Reconciliation, Anointing, Communion.

After death, the priest/minister often joins the family for prayers of commendation. Anyone may prepare the body for burial/cremation. Black is generally the colour of mourning.

Hinduism

With its complicated system of castes and sub-castes, and sects and sub-sects, Hinduism embraces wide differences in customs and rituals. Rituals sometimes differ in the same caste and sub-caste, depending on which part of India the family comes from.

Bathing early each morning in running water is important to many Hindus; very ill patients will need help if they want to continue this. Devout Hindus require time for meditation and prayer, typically at sunrise and sunset. People from certain castes prefer to die on the floor near Mother Earth.[20] When death seems imminent, a member of the family will place water on the lips of the dying person and, if possible, into the mouth as well. Many families keep a stock of water from the holy river Ganges for this purpose.

After death, the relatives should be asked about washing the body; often they want to do this themselves. Official mourning lasts 7–41 days; generally the whole extended family and friends are involved.

Islam

Prayer five times a day, preceded by washing is important. When a Muslim is dying, friends may read from the Qur'an and whisper the Muslim articles of faith in order to bring peace to the soul.[21] The whole family feel bound to visit as often as possible.

The body should *not* be washed by the hospital staff. Disposable gloves should be used for Last Offices. The right arm is placed on top of the left across the lower chest (the prayer position). The head is turned to the right and the bed moved so that the deceased faces Mecca. A Muslim undertaker, or family members of the same sex as the deceased, attend to the washing of the body.

Judaism

The local Jewish community generally organises a group of people to care for Jewish patients in hospital. Some members of the family or the community may wish to remain in the hospital with the body after death. After death, it is advisable for staff to wear disposable gloves so that there is no direct contact with the body. Members of the Jewish community will probably wash and prepare the body for burial.

Relatives are encouraged to express their grief openly, 3 days of intense grief, followed by grieving periods of 7 days and 30 days for re-adjustment. The Jewish community is very supportive during this time.

Sikhism

Founded in the fifteenth century AD as a monotheistic off-shoot of Hinduism. Sikhism is a society in which every member works for the common good. Sikh means disciple, and most come from the Punjab. There are no priests. Smoking is expressly forbidden. When close to death, the relevant part of the Sikh scriptures are read. Sikh hymns are read over the dead body in the home.

There is no objection to staff handling the body after death, but the family will generally want to wash the body themselves. White is the colour of mourning; official mourning lasts about 10 days and concludes with a special ceremony.

Bereavement
(Marilyn Relf)

> '"Mourning [grieving] is not forgetting" he said gently, his helplessness vanishing and his voice becoming wise. "It is an undoing. Every minute tie has to be untied and something permanent and valuable recovered and assimilated from the knot. The end is gain, of course. Blessed are they that mourn,[22] for they shall be made strong, in fact. But the process is like all other human births, painful and long and dangerous."'[23]

> 'An affliction of the heart may be physical as well as spiritual. Always it is the whole person who must be healed, for what hurts one part hurts the whole.'[24]

Bereavement is the greatest personal crisis that many people ever have to face and, like other stressful life events, has serious health consequences for a substantial minority of people.[25] Grief is not just emotional; it is also a behavioural, cognitive, physical, social, and spiritual experience.[26] Grief affects feelings, thoughts and behaviours (Table 2.2). A major loss forces people to adapt their assumptions about the world and of themselves and grief is a transitional process.[27] Grief is the process by which people assimilate the reality of their loss and find a way of living without the external presence of the deceased.

Social norms

Although grief is universal, the way it is experienced and expressed varies across cultures.[28] People in societies such as the UK and USA are encouraged to value self-reliance, independence and autonomy. Revealing feelings is

Table 2.2 Common reactions to bereavement

Manifestation	Description
Emotional	
Depression	Episodic waves of dejection, sadness, sorrow, despair
Anxiety	Fear of breaking down, going crazy, dying, not coping
Guilt	About events surrounding loss or past behaviour
Anger	Anger/irritability with deceased, family, friends, carers, God
Loneliness	Feeling alone, bouts of intense loneliness
Loss of enjoyment	Nothing can be pleasurable without the deceased
Relief	Relief now the suffering of the deceased has ended
Behavioural	
Agitation	Tension, restlessness, over-activity, searching for deceased
Fatigue	Cognitive impairment, lassitude, poor concentration
Crying	Tears, sad expression
Attitudes	
Self-reproach	Regrets about past behaviour toward deceased
Low self-esteem	Inadequacy, failure, incompetence, worthlessness
Hopelessness	Loss of purpose, apathy, no desire to go on living
Sense of unreality	Feeling removed from current events
Suspicion	Doubting others
Social withdrawal	Difficulty in maintaining relationships
Toward deceased	Yearning/pining, pre-occupation, hallucinations, idealisation
Physiological	
Appetite	Loss of appetite, weight change
Sleep	Insomnia, early morning waking
Physical complaints	Including headaches, muscular pains, indigestion, shortness of breath, blurred vision, lump in throat, sighing, dry mouth, palpitations, hair loss
Substance use	Increased use of psychotropic medicines, alcohol, tobacco
Illness	Particularly infections and stress-related illness

equated to weakness, and bereaved people experience social pressure to suppress emotions and hide distress, particularly men. However, these norms influence the behaviour of both men and women.[26,29] The prevailing norm is to keep grief private.[30] Bereaved people may feel both isolated and find it hard to seek help. One advantage of palliative care is that support can be offered to bereaved people without them having to seek help.

Models of grief

Models of grief provide frameworks for understanding what bereaved people tell us about their experiences. Traditionally grief has been described as a process divided into a series of overlapping phases, stages or tasks.[31,32] A central notion is that grief must be confronted and expressed, otherwise it may become pathological and manifest in some other way, such as depression or anxiety. More recent theoretical developments emphasise individual diversity.

Traditional model

Numbness
The initial reaction is shock and disbelief accompanied by feelings of unreality, and bereaved people may feel as if they are on 'automatic pilot'. Somatic symptoms may be evident.

Separation and pain

> 'The absence of the dead person is everywhere palpable. The home and family environs seem full of painful reminders. Grief breaks over the bereaved in waves of distress. There is intense yearning, as if the dead person has been torn out of his body.'[31]

Numbness gradually gives way to episodes of intense pining interspersed with periods of anxiety, tension, anger and self-reproach. The desire to recover the deceased is strong and characterised by restless searching, dreams, auditory and sensory awareness of the deceased and a pre-occupation with memories. The events surrounding the death are obsessively reviewed. Somatic symptoms are common.

Despair
Despair sets in when it is realised that the lost person will not return. Poor concentration, apathy, social withdrawal, lack of purpose and extreme sadness become common.

Acceptance
Despair gradually gives way to an acceptance of the loss. Intellectual acceptance of the finality of the loss comes first. Depression and emotional swings may continue for more than a year after bereavement.

Resolution and re-organisation
Adapting to life without the deceased includes rebuilding identity and purpose, acquiring new skills and taking on new roles. Gradually, bereaved people manage these adjustments more effectively and more positive feelings emerge. Energy returns and new interests and relationships may be developed. Eventually, bereaved people are able to remember the deceased without being overwhelmed by emotion, although anniversaries and special days may continue to trigger episodes of grief.

Unfortunately, phase models have often been interpreted as suggesting that bereavement proceeds from one clearly identifiable reaction to another in an orderly fashion. This is misleading, and these models should be used with care to avoid inappropriate behaviour towards bereaved people, such as hasty judgements as to where individuals are, or ought to be, in their grief. Accumulating evidence from empirical studies shows that grief is more complex and that people vary in the way they perceive, experience, express and cope with bereavement. Phase models provide useful descriptions of the major themes of grief.

Continuing bonds model

Successful adjustment does not depend on severing attachment to the deceased. Studies of childhood and parental grief show that attachment bonds are not relinquished but that new connections to the deceased are constructed over time.[33] Important relationships continue to influence present reality whether the person is physically present or not. This means that there may not be a definite end point that marks 'recovery' or 'closure'.

Dual process model[34]

Most people cope by oscillating between confronting grief (e.g. thinking about the deceased, pining, holding onto memories, expressing feelings) and seeking distraction in order to manage everyday life (e.g. suppressing memories and taking 'time off' from grief by keeping busy, regulating emotions). These are described as loss-oriented and restoration-oriented behaviour (Figure 2.2). Restoration-orientation enables people to undertake tasks and roles performed by the deceased, make lifestyle adjustments and build a new identity. As daily living is full of reminders of all that has been lost, people oscillate between the two ways of coping. Personality factors, gender and cultural background will influence the dominant mode and the degree to which each individual oscillates. Bereaved people are more likely to manifest loss-oriented behaviour in the early months of bereavement but in order to cope with daily life, some restoration-oriented behaviour is necessary. Thus a person may appear to be coping well one day and full of grief the next. Difficulties may emerge if the balance of behaviour is oriented exclusively on loss (chronic grief) or on restoration (absent grief).

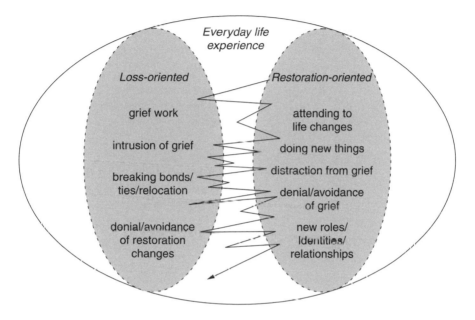

Figure 2.2 A dual process model of coping with loss. Reproduced with permission from Stroebe M and Schut H (1999).[34]

Personality has a major influence on the experience and expression of grief.[26] People who are primarily in touch with their feelings experience grief as described in the traditional models. However, people who are primarily thinkers experience grief as a cognitive process. They cope by seeking information, thinking through problems, taking action and seeking diversion. This pattern of grief is not problematic.[26] As always, it is important to enable people to build on their strengths while helping them to develop their own coping strategies.

Multidimensional models

Multidimensional models recognise loss as a process of simultaneous change and adjustment affecting many dimensions of life.[35,36] These models focus on the individual nature of each person's grief (Table 2.3) and are used widely as a framework for intervention by bereavement services.[36] Emphasis is placed on recognising that people have strengths and resources that help them to cope with bereavement.

Table 2.3   Dimensions of loss[37]

Dimension	Description
Emotional Emotional reactions	How at ease is the individual with his/her emotional responses? Do they prefer to control or express emotions?
Social Social context in which loss is experienced	How is the social network responding? What changes in status or role are being negotiated?
Physical Physical responses	Has physical health been affected?
Lifestyle Major changes, e.g. moving home, coping with single parenthood	What lifestyle changes has loss caused?
Practical Coping with everyday practicalities, e.g. cooking, shopping, self-care, child-care, housework	How is the individual managing?
Spiritual Spiritual beliefs provide meaning and purpose	How supportive is the spiritual/ religious frame of reference? Are beliefs being questioned? What meaning has been ascribed to the loss?
Identity Identity, self-esteem, self-worth	How is loss affecting concept of self?

Sources of help

Bereaved people frequently increase their use of healthcare, particularly general practitioners. Often they are seeking information and re-assurance that their grief is normal. It is good practice to give bereaved people written information about grief and local sources of help. This may be provided by local branches of national voluntary organisations such as Cruse, Bereavement Care, and the Compassionate Friends, or by church groups and the growing number of children's bereavement services, such as Winston's Wish and SeeSaw (see p.53).

Risk assessment in bereavement

'Statistical studies confirm that secure people whose experience of life has led to a reasonable trust in themselves and others will cope well with anticipated bereavements, provided they are well supported by a family who respects their need to grieve. However, multiple or unexpected and untimely losses of people on whom one depends or who depended on the survivor can overwhelm the most secure person, and lack of security and support can undermine a person's capacity to cope.'[38]

People vary enormously in their response to bereavement. Grief may be:

- immediate or delayed
- brief or seem unending
- severe or mild.

Most people work through their grief with the help of family and friends. A significant minority suffer prolonged impairment of their physical and psychological health. Bereavement is associated with health risks and:

- predisposes people to physical and mental illness
- precipitates illness and death
- exacerbates existing illness
- leads to, or exacerbates, health-threatening behaviour such as smoking, drinking and drug use
- results in an increased use in health services
- may lead to depression.[39]

A number of factors are associated with ongoing poor health. These may be identified at the time of bereavement and can be used to focus resources in order to prevent or ameliorate 'complicated' grief.[38]

Mode of death

- was it timely or untimely?
- was it expected or unexpected?
- was it unduly disturbing for the relatives or key carers?

Deaths which are untimely, unexpected and/or unduly disturbing are likely to cause more severe and more prolonged grief. Note: the death of someone with terminal illness can still be unexpected and distressing.

Nature of the relationship

How ambivalent is the relationship between key carer and patient? In a highly ambivalent relationship there is likely to be a more difficult bereavement. Often this manifests as persistent guilt feelings.

How necessary was the deceased for the key carer's sense of wellbeing, self-esteem or security? The more dependent the relationship the more all pervading the sense of loss.

Perceived support

- is the bereaved person able to share her feelings with family and friends?
- does she feel supported or isolated in her loss?

Anticipatory grieving

- were the family and patient able to talk about the illness, share feelings, and make plans for the future before the patient died?

Periods of denial by both patient and family are normal during a terminal illness but an excessive use of denial may make it harder for the survivor to start sharing with others after the patient's death.

Anger also may impede the process of grief. Angry people may deflect support and find themselves isolated.

Concurrent life events

- how much stress is the key carer/family currently facing?
    financial
    menopause
    children leaving home
    unemployment
    retirement

- how many people are dependent on the key carer, e.g. children or elderly relatives?
- has she time and space to grieve?

Previous losses

- how has the person grieved in the past?
- will the new loss uncover unresolved loss?

Medical history

- has the person a concurrent physical or psychological illness which is likely to be exacerbated by the loss?
- is there a history of alcoholism, drug abuse or suicidal behaviour?

The most positive factor in favour of a good outcome is a supportive family and/or friends who allow the bereaved person to express grief and to talk unconditionally about feelings for as long as is needed.[40]

Children and bereavement
(Ann Couldrick, Christine Pentland)

'A child can live through anything provided they are told the truth and allowed to share the natural feelings people have when they are suffering.'[41]

Every day in the UK, more than 50 children and young people under 18 are bereaved of a parent; a total of nearly 20 000 every year. By the age of 18, 7% of young people will have experienced the death of a parent.[42]

In recent years, support services for bereaved children have been established in many parts of the UK, notably Winston's Wish in Gloucestershire (www. winstonswish.org.uk).[43]

Guidance for adults about finding out if bereaved children want to see the body of their dead parent or attend the funeral is available from SeeSaw, the support service for bereaved children in Oxfordshire (www.see-saw.org.uk).

The effect of bereavement on children

Studies suggest that children are most deeply affected by:

- adverse changes in their social and financial situation (most likely if the main breadwinner dies)
- the significance of their relationship with the remaining parent
- the emotional climate in which they are helped to come to terms with their loss.

Other major factors which may affect a child include:

- bewilderment because clear information has not been given to them
- the inability of the grieving parent to respond to the needs of the child
- other adults who take on the dead parent's role
- a new home and a new school
- new roles, responsibilities and routines which adversely affect a child's sense of security
- the surviving parent remarries before the child fully understands that the dead parent will not return
- leaving their home and going to live with relatives or foster parents.

Bereaved children can adjust normally, and often do. However, disturbances in behaviour may manifest,[44] sometimes only after several months. Adults frequently do not know what to expect and may deny that a child is affected. They are often unable to perceive or respond to the very clear signals of the child's distress, even though the child may be reflecting the suppressed grief of the rest of the family.

Physical responses

- lethargy or exhaustion
- insomnia and bad dreams, or retreating into sleep as an escape
- loss of appetite, compulsive eating, craving certain foods
- regression to urinary and/or faecal incontinence
- rashes, fever, nausea
- exacerbation of asthma, eczema or other pre-existing condition
- in an older child, symptoms may mimic those of the dead person.

Emotional responses

- panic attacks and/or increased anxiety, often resulting in the child not wanting to leave home or go to school
- becoming more clinging and dependent

- exaggerated separation responses, e.g. intense distress when the surviving parent walks out of the room or leaves for short periods
- rapid mood swings from being all right and happy to weeping, depression, rejection of carer(s), withdrawal, or inappropriately aggressive responses
- guilt, i.e. child believing that something they said or did contributed to the death.

Cognitive effects

- poor concentration resulting in difficulties at school
- loss of short-term and/or long-term memory
- poor motivation, e.g. 'What's the point of anything now?'
- learning difficulties, the nature of which will depend upon the child's developmental stage.

Behavioural responses

- anxiety about or dislike of change in routine(s)
- regression, e.g. wanting to be fed, or rocked in the surviving parent's arms
- behaviour reflecting an unconscious and often aggressive response, e.g. playing very loud music, dangerous competitive activities such as racing bikes or cars, and stealing
- putting on a brave face for the sake of the surviving parent, or because of a fear of losing control.

Approach the parent as a colleague

Remember, parents have expert knowledge about their children. Boost confidence and increase their feelings of competence by:

- explaining the physical, emotional, cognitive and behavioural changes which may occur and assure parents that these are normal reactions for children
- recommending appropriate books and leaflets; these help some parents to gain intellectual mastery over the situation (Box 2.C)
- suggesting that parents encourage children to draw, paint or write about their experience of the loss and to talk about the implications
- suggesting that the children are encouraged to make a scrapbook of memories, e.g. photos, cards, letters, and collecting mementos and talking about these
- warning parents that young children's play and interests may appear to revolve around dying, death and funerals; this is a natural way for children

---

Box 2.C   Examples of helpful reading material

When a parent becomes seriously ill
For parents:
Winston's Wish (2001) *As Big As It Gets.*

For primary school children:
Stokes J and Bailey P (2000) *The Secret C.* Winston's Wish.

When a parent dies
For primary school children:
Varley S (1985) *Badger's Parting Gifts* (2e). Harper Collins, London.
Thomas P (2000) *I Miss You – a first look at death.* Hodder Wayland, London.

An activity book for young children:
Crossley D and Sheppard K (2000) *Muddles, Puddles and Sunshine.* Hawthorn Press, Stroud.

For teenagers:
Krementz J (1983) *How It Feels When A Parent Dies.* Gollancz, London.
Abrams R (1999) *When Parents Die.* Routledge, London.

Details of additional reading material can be obtained from Winston's Wish (www.winstonswish.org.uk) or SeeSaw (www.see-saw.org.uk).

---

to work through their distress and gain a greater understanding of what has happened
- warning parents that some children try to ignore the loss, and to behave and play as if nothing significant has happened
- telling parents not to be too hard on themselves; it is normal sometimes to shout at and be impatient with children
- encouraging parents to be open with the children about how they are feeling themselves; in doing this, parents are modelling the honest expression of feelings
    'I'm crying because I am sad'
    'I'm angry because we cannot do that together again'
    'I'm laughing because I am remembering how funny it was when ...'
- encouraging parents to involve others (relatives, friends, teachers) for both practical help and emotional support
- being aware of and sensitive to the family's belief and value systems; do not impose your own, and avoid 'ought' and 'should'
- encouraging parents to look after their own physical, practical and emotional needs; if they do, parents will be better able to deal with their children's needs and demands (Box 2.D).

Box 2.D A charter for bereaved children created by Winston's Wish (1998), a community-based bereavement programme for children, young people and their families in Gloucestershire, UK

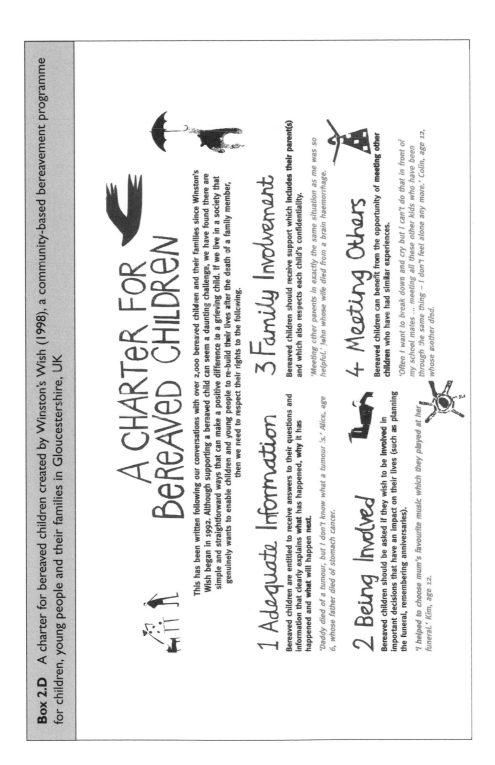

A CHARTER FOR BEREAVED CHILDREN

This has been written following our conversations with over 2,000 bereaved children and their families since Winston's Wish began in 1992. Although supporting a bereaved child can seem a daunting challenge, we have found there are simple and straightforward ways that can make a positive difference to a grieving child. If we live in a society that genuinely wants to enable children and young people to re-build their lives after the death of a family member, then we need to respect their rights to the following.

1 Adequate Information

Bereaved children are entitled to receive answers to their questions and information that clearly explains what has happened, why it has happened and what will happen next.

'Daddy died of a tumour, but I don't know what a tumour 'is.' Alice, age 6, whose father died of stomach cancer.

2 Being Involved

Bereaved children should be asked if they wish to be involved in important decisions that have an impact on their lives (such as planning the funeral, remembering anniversaries).

'I helped to choose mum's favourite music which they played at her funeral.' Kim, age 12.

3 Family Involvement

Bereaved children should receive support which includes their parent(s) and which also respects each child's confidentiality.

'Meeting other parents in exactly the same situation as me was so helpful.' John whose wife died from a brain haemorrhage.

4 Meeting Others

Bereaved children can benefit from the opportunity of meeting other children who have had similar experiences.

'Often I want to break down and cry but I can't do that in front of my school mates ... meeting all these other kids who have been through the same thing – I don't feel alone any more.' Colin, age 12, whose mother died.

5 Telling the Story

Bereaved children have a right to tell their story in a variety of ways and for those stories to be heard, read or seen by those important to them. For example, through drawing, puppets, letters and words.

'My picture shows the car banged dad on the head, he fell off his bike, hit his head and died later in hospital.' Georgina, age 7, whose father died in a road accident.

6 Expressing Feelings

Bereaved children should feel comfortable expressing all feelings associated with grief, such as anger, sadness, guilt and anxiety, and to be helped to find appropriate ways to do this.

'It's alright to cry and OK to be happy as well.' James, aged 9, whose dad died from a heart attack.

7 Not to Blame

Bereaved children should be helped to understand they are not responsible and not to blame for the death.

'I now understand it wasn't anyone's fault.' Chris, age 12, whose dad died by suicide.

8 Established Routines

Bereaved children should be able to choose to continue previously enjoyed activities and interests.

'I went to Brownies after Meg died. I wanted my friends to know.'

9 School Response

Bereaved children can benefit from receiving an appropriate and positive response from their school or college.

'My teacher remembers the days which are difficult, like Father's Day and dad's birthday.' Alex, age 9.

10 Remembering

Bereaved children have a right to remember the person who has died for the rest of their lives if they wish to do so. This may involve re-living memories (both good and difficult) so that the person becomes a comfortable part of the child's on-going life story.

'I like to show my memory book to people who didn't have the chance to know my dad.' Bethany, age 8, whose father died from cancer.

References

1   Simpson M (1979) *The Facts of Death*. Prentice-Hall, Englewood Cliffs, NJ.
2   Johnson J (1987) Supplied by Hunkin V (personal communication).
3   Maguire P (1999) *Communication Skills for Doctors*. Arnold, London.
4   Parkes CM (1972) Accuracy of predictions of survival in later stages of cancer. *British Medical Journal.* **2:** 29–33.
5   Massie M and Holland J (1989) Overview of normal reactions and prevalence of psychiatric disorders. In: J Holland and J Rowland (eds) *Handbook of Psychooncology.* Oxford University Press, Oxford, pp 273–282.
6   Hotopf M *et al.* (2002) Depression in advanced disease: a systematic review Part 1. Prevalence and case finding. *Palliative Medicine.* **16:** 81–97.
7   Maguire P and Faulkner A (1993) Handling the withdrawn patient – a flow diagram. *Palliative Medicine.* **7:** 333–338.
8   Mayne M (1995) *This Sunrise of Wonder.* Fount, London, p. 21.
9   Spiritual Care WG (1994) *Spiritual Care Working Group.* Sir Michael Sobell House, Oxford.
10 Edassery D and Kutticrath S (1998) Spirituality in the secular sense. *European Journal of Palliative Care.* **5:** 165–167.
11 Kubotera T (1988) Personal communication.
12 Sulmasy D (1997) *The Healer's Calling. A spirituality for physicians and other health care professionals.* Paulist Press, New York, pp 55–70.
13 Rousseau P (2000) Spirituality and the dying patient. *Journal of Clinical Oncology.* **18:** 2000–2002.
14 Speck P (1984) *Being There: pastoral care in time of illness.* SPCK, London.
15 Hamilton D (1998) Believing in patients' beliefs: physician attunement to the spiritual dimension as a positive factor in patient healing and health. *American Journal of Hospice and Palliative Care.* **15:** 276–279.
16 Morgan P and Lawton C (1996) *Ethical Issues in Six Religious Traditions.* Edinburgh University Press, Edinburgh.
17 Neuberger J (1993) *Caring for Dying People of Different Faiths.* Midwives Press.
18 Rinpoche S (1992) *The Tibetan Book of Living and Dying.* Harper Press, San Francisco, pp 90–92.
19 Green J (1989) Buddhism. *Nursing Times.* **85:** 40–41.
20 Green J (1989) Hinduism. *Nursing Times.* **85:** 50–51.
21 Gatrad A (1994) Muslim customs surrounding death, bereavement, postmortem examinations, and organ transplants. *British Medical Journal.* **309:** 521–523.
22 Grieve R and Dixon P (1983) Dysphagia: a further symptom of hypercalcaemia. *British Medical Journal.* **286:** 1935–1936.
23 Allingham M (1957) *The Tiger in the Smoke.* Penguin, Harmondsworth.
24 Campbell A (1987) Quote. In: D O'Toole (ed) *Healing and Growing Through Grief.* Blue Cross and Blue Shield, Michigan.
25 Stroebe W and Stroebe M (1987) *Bereavement and Health.* Cambridge University Press, Cambridge.
26 Martin T and Doka K (2000) *Men Don't Cry ... Women Do.* Taylor and Francis, Philadelphia.
27 Parkes C (1993) Bereavement as a psychosocial transition: processes of adaptation to change. In: M Stroebe *et al.* (eds) *Handbook of Bereavement.* Cambridge University Press, Cambridge, pp 91–101.
28 Parkes C *et al.* (1997) *Death and Bereavement Across Cultures.* Routledge, London.
29 Riches G and Dawson P (2000) *An Intimate Loneliness.* Open University Press, Buckingham.
30 Walter T (1999) *On Bereavement: the culture of grief.* Open University Press, Buckingham.
31 Parkes C (1986) *Bereavement: studies of grief in adult life.* Pelican, London.
32 Worden J (1991) *Grief Counselling and Grief Therapy.* Tavistock, London.

33 Klass D *et al.* (1996) *Continuing Bonds.* Taylor and Francis, Washington.
34 Stroebe M and Schut H (1999) The dual process model of coping with bereavement; rationale and description. *Death Studies.* **23:** 197–224.
35 Shuchter S and Zisook S (1993) The course of normal grief. In: M Stroebe *et al.* (eds) *Handbook of Bereavement.* Cambridge University Press, Cambridge, pp 23–43.
36 Parkes CM *et al.* (1996) *Counselling in Terminal Care and Bereavement.* British Psychological Society, Leicester.
37 Payne S *et al.* (1999) *Loss and Bereavement.* Open University Press, Buckingham.
38 Parkes C (1990) Risk factors in bereavement: implications for the prevention and treatment of pathologic grief. *Psychiatric Annals.* **20:** 308–313.
39 Osterweiss M *et al.* (1984) *Bereavement Reactions: consequences and care.* National Academy Press, Washington.
40 Raphael B (1977) Preventive intervention with the recently bereaved. *Archives of General Psychiatry.* **34:** 1450–1454.
41 LeShan E. Source unknown.
42 Winston's Wish (2002) Unpublished material.
43 Stokes J *et al.* (1999) Developing services for bereaved children: a discussion of the theoretical and practical issues involved. *Mortality.* **4:** 291–307.
44 Dowdney L *et al.* (1999) Psychological disturbance and service provision in parentally bereaved children: prospective case-control study. *British Medical Journal.* **319:** 354–357.

PART THREE

Symptom management I

General principles · Pain · Pain management
Use of analgesics · Non-opioid (antipyretic) analgesics
Weak opioid analgesics · Strong opioid analgesics
Adjuvant analgesics · Alternative routes of administration

General principles

The scientific approach to symptom management can be encapsulated in the acronym '**EFMMA**':

- Evaluation: *diagnosis of each symptom before treatment*
- Explanation: *explanation to the patient before treatment*
- Management: *individualised treatment*
- Monitoring: *continuing review of the impact of treatment*
- Attention to detail: *no unwarranted assumptions.*

Evaluation

Evaluation must always precede treatment.

Evaluation is based on *probability* and *pattern recognition*.

Patients may be reluctant to bother their doctor about symptoms such as dry mouth, altered taste, anorexia, pruritus and insomnia. Enquiries should be made from time to time rather than relying entirely on spontaneous reports.

What is the cause of the symptom?

The cancer is not always the cause of a symptom. Causal factors also include:

- treatment
- debility
- concurrent disorders.

Some symptoms are caused by several factors. All symptoms are made worse by insomnia, exhaustion, anxiety, fear, helplessness, hopelessness, and depression.

What is the underlying pathological mechanism?

Even when the cancer is responsible, a symptom may be caused by different mechanisms, e.g. vomiting from hypercalcaemia and from raised intracranial pressure. Treatment varies accordingly.

What has been tried and failed?

This helps in planning the most appropriate management strategy by excluding certain treatment options, provided they were used optimally. If not, a further trial of a given drug may be indicated.

What is the impact of the symptom on the patient's life?

The following questions help to determine how big an impact a symptom is having on the patient's life:

'How much does [the symptom] affect your life?'
'What makes it worse and what makes it better?'
'Is it worse at any particular time of the day or night?'
'Does it disturb your sleep at all?'

Explanation

Explain the underlying mechanism(s) in simple terms

Treatment begins with an explanation by the doctor of the reason(s) for the symptom, for example, 'The shortness of breath is caused partly by the cancer itself and partly by fluid at the base of the right lung. In addition, you are anaemic'. This knowledge often does much to reduce the negative psychological impact of the symptom, and thereby reduces the severity of the symptom itself.

If explanation is omitted, patients continue to think that their condition is shrouded in mystery. This is frightening because 'even the doctors don't know what's going on'. Explanation generally enables patients to see more clearly the rationale behind any suggested treatment, thereby improving compliance.

Discuss treatment options with the patient

Whenever possible, the doctor and the patient should decide together on the immediate course of action. Few things are more damaging to a person's self-esteem than to be excluded from discussions about one's self.

Management

Correct the correctable

Palliative care includes disorder-specific treatment when it is practical and not disproportionately burdensome. For example, patients with breathlessness and bronchospasm benefit from bronchodilator therapy. Likewise, aqueous cream applied topically will moisturise dry skin, and thereby relieve pruritus.

Use non-drug as well as drug treatments

Examples of non-drug treatment are contained in the sections dealing with individual symptoms. Relaxation therapy is an example of a non-drug treatment with wide applicability.

Prescribe drugs prophylactically for persistent symptoms

When treating a persistent symptom with a drug, it should be administered regularly 'by the clock' on a prophylactic basis. The use of drugs as needed (p.r.n.) instead of regularly is the cause of much unrelieved distress.

Keep the treatment as straightforward as possible

When an additional drug is considered, ask the following questions:

'What is the treatment goal?'
'How can it be monitored?'
'What is the risk of undesirable effects?'
'What is the risk of drug interactions?'
'Is it possible to stop any of the current medications?'

Written advice is essential

Precise guidelines are necessary to achieve maximum patient co-operation. 'Take as much as you like, as often as you like' is a recipe for anxiety, poor symptom relief and maximum undesirable effects. The drug regimen should be written out in full for the patient and his family to work from. Times to be taken, names of drugs, reason for use (for pain, for bowels, etc.) and dose (x ml, y tablets) should all be stated. Also the patient should be advised how to obtain further supplies (generally from their general practitioner).

Seek a colleague's advice in seemingly intractable situations

No one is an expert in all aspects of patient care. For example, the management of an unusual genito-urinary problem is likely to be enhanced by advice from a urologist or gynaecologist.

Never say 'I have tried everything' or 'There's nothing more that I can do'

It is generally possible to develop a repertoire of measures. Without promising too much, assure the patient that you are going to do all you can to help, e.g. 'No promises but we'll do our best'.

Often it is a case of chipping away at symptoms, a little at a time, and not expecting immediate, complete relief. When tackled in this way it is surprising how much can be achieved with determination and persistence.

Monitoring

Review! Review! Review!

Patients vary and it is not always possible to predict the optimum dose of opioids, laxatives and psychotropic drugs. Undesirable effects put drug compliance in jeopardy. Arrangements must be made for monitoring and adjusting medication. Further, cancer is a progressive disease, and new symptoms occur. These must be dealt with urgently.

It may be necessary to compromise on complete relief in order to avoid unacceptable undesirable effects. For example, antimuscarinic effects such as dry mouth or visual disturbance may limit dose escalation and, with inoperable bowel obstruction, it may be better to reduce vomiting to once or twice a day rather than seeking complete relief.

Attention to detail

Attention to detail makes all the difference to palliative care; without it success may be forfeited and patients suffer needlessly. Attention to detail requires an inquisitive mind, one which repeatedly asks 'Why?'

> 'Why is this patient with breast cancer vomiting? She's not taking morphine; she's not hypercalcaemic. Why is she vomiting?'
> 'This patient with cancer of the pancreas has pain in the neck. It does not fit with the typical pattern of metastatic spread. Why does he have pain there?'

It is important not to make unwarranted assumptions. Remember: to *ass-u-me* means to make an *ass* of *u* and *me*.[1]

Attention to detail is important at every stage: in evaluation, explanation (avoid jargon, use simple language), when deciding management (e.g. drug regimens which are easy to follow, providing written advice) and when monitoring treatment. Attention to detail is equally important in relation to the non-physical aspects of care. All symptoms are exaggerated by negative emotions, e.g. anxiety and fear.

Pain

> *'Pain is what the patient says hurts.'*

Pain is an unpleasant *sensory* and *emotional* experience associated with actual or potential tissue damage or described in terms of such damage.[2] In other words, pain is a *somatopsychic* phenomenon and is modulated by:

- the patient's *mood*
- the patient's *morale*
- the *meaning* of the pain for the patient.

The meaning of persistent pain in advanced cancer is, 'I am incurable; I am going to die'. Various factors affecting pain intensity are shown in Box 3.A. Because pain is multidimensional, it is helpful to think in terms of *total pain*, encompassing physical, psychological, social and spiritual aspects of suffering (Figure 3.1).

Box 3.A   Factors affecting pain intensity

Pain increased	Pain decreased
Discomfort	Relief of other symptoms
Insomnia	Sleep
Fatigue	Understanding
Anxiety	Companionship
Fear	Creative activity
Anger	Relaxation
Sadness	Reduction in anxiety
Depression	Elevation of mood
Boredom	Analgesics
Mental isolation	Anxiolytics
Social abandonment	Antidepressants

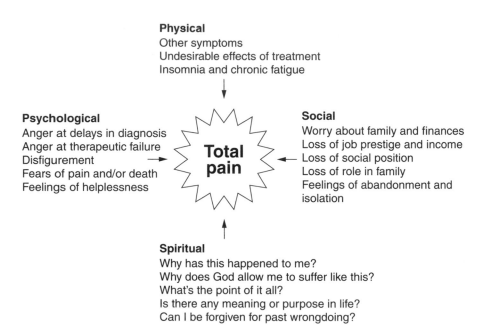

Physical
Other symptoms
Undesirable effects of treatment
Insomnia and chronic fatigue

Psychological
Anger at delays in diagnosis
Anger at therapeutic failure
Disfigurement
Fears of pain and/or death
Feelings of helplessness

Total pain

Social
Worry about family and finances
Loss of job prestige and income
Loss of social position
Loss of role in family
Feelings of abandonment and isolation

Spiritual
Why has this happened to me?
Why does God allow me to suffer like this?
What's the point of it all?
Is there any meaning or purpose in life?
Can I be forgiven for past wrongdoing?

Figure 3.1   The four dimensions of pain.

People with chronic pain generally do not look in pain because of the absence of autonomic concomitants (Table 3.1). However, in cancer, such concomitants may be present if the pain is of recent onset, or is paroxysmal.

Table 3.1   Temporal classification of pain

	Acute		*Chronic*
Time course	Transient		Persistent
Meaning to patient	Positive draws attention to injury or illness	Negative serves no useful purpose	Positive as patient obtains secondary gain
Concomitants	Fight or flight pupillary dilation increased sweating tachypnoea tachycardia shunting of blood from viscera to muscles		Vegetative sleep disturbance anorexia decreased libido no pleasure in life constipation somatic pre-occupation personality change lethargy

Pain management

Evaluation

Pain and advanced cancer are not synonymous:

- 3/4 of patients experience pain
- 1/4 of patients do not experience pain.

Multiple concurrent pains are common in those who have pain. Approximately:

- 1/3 has a single pain
- 1/3 has two pains
- 1/3 has three or more pains.[3]

Evaluation is a multidimensional process, partly synchronous and partly sequential (Figure 3.2). It begins by asking the patient to identify the *location* of the pain ('Where exactly is your pain?') and its *duration* ('When did it start?'). Then while the patient goes on to describe the pain, the doctor reflects on:

- the cause of the pain (cancer vs non-cancer)
- the underlying mechanism (pathological vs functional)
- the contribution of non-physical factors.

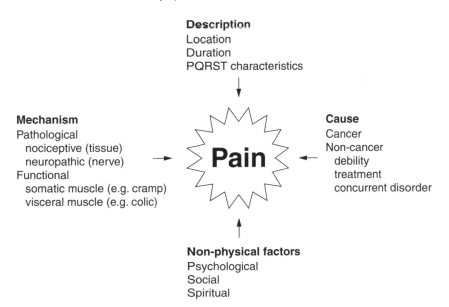

Figure 3.2 The four dimensions of pain evaluation.

The patient's description of her pain may need to be prompted by a series of questions about the PQRST characteristics of pain (Box 3.B).

Box 3.B   The PQRST characteristics of pain

Palliative factors	'What makes it better?'
Provocative factors	'What makes it worse?'
Quality	'What exactly is it like?'
Radiation	'Does it spread anywhere?'
Severity	'How severe is it?'
	'How much does it affect your life?'
Temporal factors	'Is it there all the time or does it come and go?'
	'Is it worse at any particular time of the day or night?'

In practice it may be better to begin with T and end with P, i.e. TSRQP!

Causes of pain

Pain in cancer can be grouped into four causal categories:

● *cancer*, e.g. soft tissue, visceral, bone, neuropathic
● *treatment*, e.g. chemotherapy-related mucositis
● *debility*, e.g. constipation, muscle tension/spasm
● *concurrent disorders*, e.g. spondylosis, osteo-arthritis.

In 15% of patients with advanced cancer and pain, none of their pain is caused by the cancer itself.[3]

Mechanisms of pain

It is important to distinguish between *functional* and *pathological* pains. Functional muscle pains are part of everybody's general life experience and are common in patients with advanced cancer. For example:

● somatic muscle-tension pains, e.g. tension headache, cramp, myofascial
● visceral muscle-tension pains, e.g. distension, colic.

Myofascial pain is a specific form of cramp related to myofascial trigger points.[4] These occur most commonly in the muscles of the pectoral girdle and neck, and are likely to be more troublesome in physically debilitated and anxious persons.

Pathological pains can be divided into:

- nociceptive (associated with tissue distortion or injury)
- neuropathic (associated with nerve compression or injury).

Pain in an area of abnormal or absent sensation is always neuropathic.

There are many causes of neuropathic pain in cancer (Box 3.C). When caused by cancer, nerve compression generally precedes nerve injury. Nerve compression manifests as a deep ache of variable intensity in a neurodermatomal distribution. The characteristics of nerve injury pain are often distinct (Box 3.D), and relate to:

- neuronal hyperexcitability and spontaneous activity at the site of injury
- a cascade of neurochemical and physiological changes in the CNS, particularly in the dorsal horn of the spinal cord ('central sensitisation').

Nerve injury does not always result in pain. With identical lesions, only a minority develops pain; a genetic factor has been postulated.

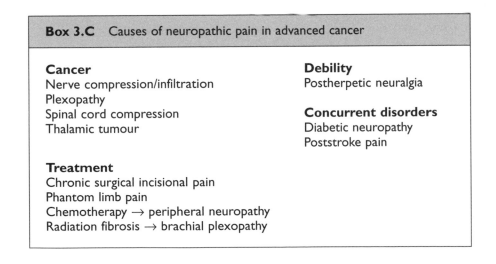

Box 3.C Causes of neuropathic pain in advanced cancer

Cancer
Nerve compression/infiltration
Plexopathy
Spinal cord compression
Thalamic tumour

Treatment
Chronic surgical incisional pain
Phantom limb pain
Chemotherapy → peripheral neuropathy
Radiation fibrosis → brachial plexopathy

Debility
Postherpetic neuralgia

Concurrent disorders
Diabetic neuropathy
Poststroke pain

Box 3.D   Clinical features of nerve injury pain

Distribution
If a peripheral nerve lesion, neurodermatomal.
If central, an area of pain within a larger area of abnormal sensation or dysfunction.

Quality
One or all of the following:
● superficial burning/stinging pain, particularly if a peripheral lesion
● spontaneous stabbing/lancinating pain
● a deep ache.

Concomitants
Often there is:
● allodynia (light touch exacerbates pain), e.g. unable to bear clothing on the affected area
● a sensory deficit, generally numbness.

Occasionally there is a sympathetic component manifesting as:
● cutaneous vasodilation → increased skin temperature
● sweating.

Patients also become exhausted and demoralised, particularly if there is insomnia.

Relief from analgesics
About 50% of nerve injury pains caused by cancer respond to the combined use of a NSAID and a strong opioid; the rest need adjuvant analgesics.[5]

Sympathetically maintained pain is an uncommon form of neuropathic pain, related to sympathetic nerve trauma at operation or 'irritation' by a tumour. Its characteristics are similar to somatic nerve injury pain except that it:

● has an arterial distribution instead of a neurodermatomal one (often not obvious)
● differs in its response to treatment (often poor response to analgesics and adjuvants).[6]

The treatment of the different types of pain is not always identical, and may be completely different (Table 3.2). If there is a sympathetic component, a regional sympathetic block may help.

Table 3.2 Mechanisms of pain and implications for treatment

Type of pain	Mechanism	Examples	Response to opioids	Typical treatment
Nociceptive	Stimulation of nerve endings			
muscle spasm		Cramp	−	Muscle relaxant
somatic		Soft tissue, bone pain	±	NSAID ± opioid
visceral		Liver capsule pain	±	Opioid ± NSAID
Neuropathic				
nerve compression	Stimulation of nervi nervorum		±	Opioid + corticosteroid (if cancer)
nerve injury	Peripheral nerve injury	Neuroma or nerve infiltration, e.g. brachial or lumbosacral plexus	±	Opioid; NSAID (if cancer); tricyclic antidepressant; anti-epileptic; NMDA-receptor-channel blocker; spinal analgesia; TENS
de-afferentation pain				
central pain	CNS injury	Spinal cord compression or poststroke pain		

Non-physical factors

Non-physical factors always influence pain intensity (Figure 3.1). Psychosocial evaluation is therefore important. The ability to facilitate a patient's fears and anxieties is crucial to success in cancer pain management. In a few patients, the help of a clinical psychologist or a psychiatrist may be necessary if the patient seems to be using pain to express otherwise inexpressible negative emotions ('somatisation').

Explanation

Given that many patients have pain which is not caused by the cancer, the positive value of an explanation of the causes and mechanisms of their pains is self-evident. In relation to neuropathic pain which is not responding to standard analgesics, it is important to tell the patient that:

- nerve compression pain 'often needs cortisone as well as painkillers'
- nerve injury pain 'sometimes does not respond to painkillers like aspirin and morphine ... Because of this we need to start a different type of pain-killer ... The first step is to get you a good night's sleep'.

Management

Pain relief often requires a broad-spectrum multimodal approach (Box 3.E). For pain caused by the cancer itself, drugs generally give adequate relief provided the right drugs are administered in the right doses at the right time intervals. It is often best to aim at progressive pain relief:

- relief at night
- relief at rest during the day
- relief on movement (not always completely possible).

If anticancer treatment is recommended, analgesics should be given until the treatment ameliorates the pain; this may take several weeks. Since the advent of spinal analgesia (*see* p.99), neurolytic and neurosurgical procedures have become almost obsolete in the UK. At many centres, coeliac axis plexus block with alcohol for epigastric visceral pain is the only neurolytic block still used.

Some patients continue to experience pain on movement despite analgesics, other drugs, radiotherapy and nerve blocks. Here, the situation is often improved by suggesting modifications to the patient's way of life and

Box 3.E   Pain management in cancer

Modification of the pathological process
Radiation therapy
Hormone therapy
Chemotherapy
Surgery

Analgesics
Non-opioid (antipyretic)
Opioid
Adjuvant
   corticosteroids
   antidepressants
   anti-epileptics
   NMDA-receptor-channel blocker
   muscle relaxants
   antispasmodics
   bisphosphonates

Non-drug methods
Physical
   massage
   massage
   heat pads
   TENS

Psychological
Relaxation
Cognitive-behavioural therapy
Psychodynamic therapy

Interruption of pain pathways
Local anaesthesia
   lidocaine
   bupivacaine
Neurolysis
   chemical, e.g. alcohol, phenol
   cryotherapy
   thermocoagulation
Neurosurgery
   cervical cordotomy

Modification of way of life and environment
Avoid pain-precipitating activities
Immobilisation of the painful part
   cervical collar
   surgical corset
   slings
   orthopaedic surgery
Walking aid
Wheelchair
Hoist

environment. The help of a physiotherapist and an occupational therapist is often invaluable.

Relief should be evaluated in relation to each pain. If there is severe anxiety and/or depression, it may take 3–4 weeks to achieve maximum benefit. Re-evaluation is a continuing necessity; old pains may get worse and new ones develop.

Use of analgesics

Analgesics can be divided into three classes:

- non-opioid (antipyretic)
- opioid
- adjuvant.

Non-opioid and opioid analgesics both act peripherally and centrally.[7,8] The principles governing analgesic use include:[9]

- *by the mouth*, the oral route is the standard route for analgesics, including morphine and other strong opioids
- *by the clock*, persistent pain requires preventive therapy. Analgesics should be given regularly and prophylactically; as needed (p.r.n.) medication alone is irrational and inhumane (Figure 3.3)
- *by the ladder*, use the analgesic ladder (Figure 3.4). If after optimising the dose a drug fails to relieve, move up the ladder, do not move sideways in the same efficacy group
- *individualised treatment*, the right dose is the one which relieves the pain; doses should be titrated upwards until the pain is relieved or undesirable effects prevent further escalation
- *use of adjuvant drugs*, in the context of the analgesic ladder these include
    other drugs which relieve pain in specific situations
    drugs to control the undesirable effects of analgesics
    concurrently prescribed psychotropic medication, e.g. anxiolytics.

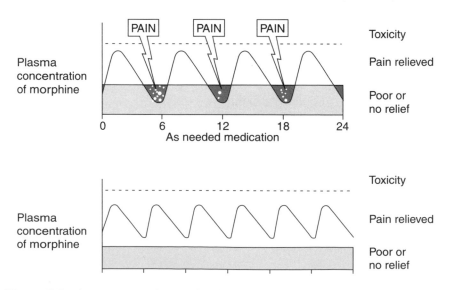

Figure 3.3   A comparison of as needed (p.r.n.) dosing and regular q4h morphine.

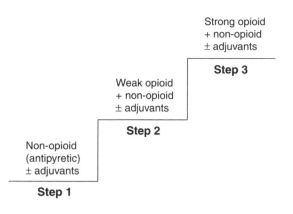

Figure 3.4 The World Health Organization analgesic ladder for cancer pain.

A key concept underlying the analgesic ladder is 'broad-spectrum analgesia', i.e. drugs from each of the three classes of analgesic are used appropriately, either singly or in combination, to maximise their impact (Figure 3.5). Relief with morphine and other opioids is often limited in the presence of central sensitisation. This occurs when there is peripheral hyperexcitability as a result of inflammation or nerve injury (Figure 3.6). This is why it is important to use a NSAID and an opioid in combination for most cancer pains, particularly bone and soft tissue pain, but also for nerve injury pain.

Non-opioid (antipyretic) analgesics

The non-opioid (antipyretic) analgesics comprise:

- paracetamol
- non-steroidal anti-inflammatory drugs (NSAIDs).

Paracetamol

Paracetamol (acetaminophen USA) is an antipyretic analgesic which inhibits cyclo-oxygenase (COX) in the CNS,[10] and interacts with several other central systems, e.g. opioidergic and serotoninergic.[11] However, although it also has a peripheral analgesic effect,[12] it does not have an anti-inflammatory effect

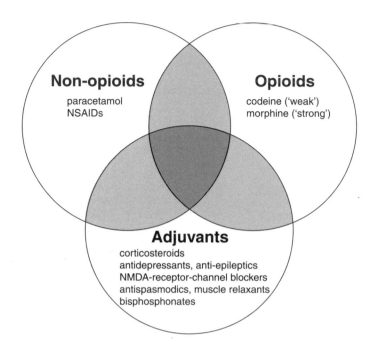

Figure 3.5   Broad-spectrum analgesia.

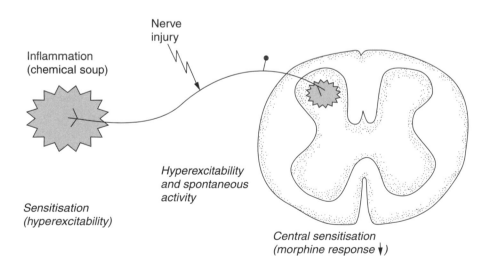

Figure 3.6   Peripheral sensitisation leads to central sensitisation and a reduced response to opioids.

in inflamed joints. The following features also distinguish paracetamol from NSAIDs:

- undesirable effects are uncommon
- does not injure the gastric mucosa, although it may cause non-specific dyspepsia
- is well tolerated by patients with peptic ulcers
- does not affect plasma uric acid concentration.

Paracetamol has no effect on platelet function. In addition, it can be taken by 2/3 of patients who are hypersensitive to aspirin.[13] NSAIDs and paracetamol can be used together with an additive effect. The main drawbacks with paracetamol are the frequency of administration, generally q6h, and its potential for hepatotoxicity.[11]

NSAIDs

NSAIDs are of particular benefit for pains associated with inflammation, e.g. soft tissue infiltration and bone metastases. Because inflammation leads to central sensitisation and increased pain, NSAIDs sometimes play a crucial role in relieving cancer-related neuropathic pain.[14]

Ibuprofen, diclofenac and naproxen are all commonly used in palliative care in the UK; flurbiprofen is the preferred NSAID at Sir Michael Sobell House. This could change now that less gastrotoxic selective COX-2 inhibitors are available (see below).

NSAIDs inhibit cyclo-oxygenase (COX), an important enzyme in the arachidonic acid cascade which results in the production of tissue and inflammatory PGs.[10] Although it appears to explain most of their undesirable effects, inhibition of PG synthesis does not account for the total analgesic effect of NSAIDs. Thus, in postdental extraction pain, most weak COX inhibitors are significantly superior to aspirin and most strong COX inhibitors are inferior.[15] Further, the central analgesic effects of NSAIDs have not been fully elucidated, and clinically important differences could still emerge.[7]

COX exists in two forms. COX-1 is present in all normal tissues (and is described as *constitutive*), whereas COX-2 is generally undetectable except when massively induced by inflammation (Figure 3.7). By using selective COX-2 inhibitors, gastric toxicity is reduced.[16,17] However, COX-1 inhibition alone does not explain the differential impact of NSAIDs on the gastro-intestinal tract; uncoupling of oxidative phosphorylation is possibly more important.[18] COX-2 is present in the kidneys in the region of the juxtaglomerular apparatus, and selective COX-2 inhibitors (like non-selective NSAIDs) can cause fluid retention and may adversely affect renal function.

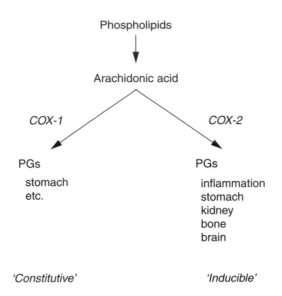

Figure 3.7 Cyclo-oxygenase (COX) and the production of prostaglandins (PGs).

NSAIDs differ in their effect on platelet function. In patients undergoing chemotherapy or with thrombocytopenia from other causes, it is best to use a NSAID which has no effect on platelet function (Table 3.3). Most NSAIDs, and sometimes paracetamol, induce bronchospasm in certain patients. *Choline salicylate, choline magnesium trisalicylate, azapropazone, nimesulide* (not available in UK) and *benzydamine (oral rinse)* do not. Meloxicam and celecoxib (COX-1 sparing NSAIDs) and rofecoxib (specific COX-2 inhibitor) are also generally safe in this respect.[19]

Note:

- aspirin may cause tinnitus and deafness, particularly in patients with a low plasma albumin
- aspirin and salicylates have a modest hypoglycaemic effect, e.g. aspirin ⩾1200mg/24h; occasionally it may be necessary to reduce the dose of insulin or oral hypoglycaemic agent[20]
- aspirin *antagonises* uricosuric agents
- all NSAIDs cause salt and water retention which may result in ankle oedema; they therefore *antagonise* the action of diuretics
- NSAIDs may cause renal failure (acute or acute-on-chronic), particularly in patients with hypovolaemia from any cause, e.g. diuretics, fever, dehydration, vomiting, diarrhoea, haemorrhage, surgery
- NSAIDs may also cause interstitial nephritis (± nephrotic syndrome or papillary necrosis); this is sporadic and unpredictable.

Table 3.3 NSAIDs and impairment of platelet function

Drug	Effect	Comment
Dual COX inhibitors		
Aspirin	+	*Irreversible* platelet dysfunction as a result of acetylation of platelet COX-1
Non-acetylated salicylates e.g. choline magnesium trisalicylate, diflunisal, salsalate	–	No effect at recommended doses
Classical NSAIDs *except diclofenac* e.g. ibuprofen, flurbiprofen, ketorolac, naproxen	+	Reversible platelet dysfunction
Diclofenac	–	Although diclofenac *in vitro* is a potent reversible inhibitor of platelet aggregation, typical oral doses of diclofenac *in vivo* do not affect platelet function[21]
COX-1 sparing NSAIDs Nimesulide,[22] celecoxib,[23] meloxicam[24]	–	
Specific COX-2 inhibitors Rofecoxib[25]	–	

Weak opioid analgesics

The division of opioids into 'weak' and 'strong' is to a certain extent arbitrary (Table 3.4). By IM injection, most weak opioids can provide analgesia equivalent, or nearly equivalent, to morphine 10mg. However, codeine, dextropropoxyphene and dihydrocodeine are not used parenterally. There is little to choose between these three opioids in terms of efficacy. Pentazocine is not recommended; it is short-acting and often causes psychotomimetic effects, e.g. hallucinations, feelings of unreality, dysphoria.

Weak opioids are said to have a ceiling effect for analgesia. This is an oversimplification; mixed agonist-antagonists such as pentazocine have a true ceiling effect but the maximum dose of a weak opioid agonist is determined by a disproportionate increase in undesirable effects, particularly nausea and

Table 3.4 Weak opioids

Drug	Bio-availability (%)	Time to maximum concentration (h)	Plasma halflife (h)	Duration of analgesia (h)[a]	Potency ratio with codeine
Codeine	40 (12–84)	1–2	2.5–3.5	4–5	1
Dextropropoxyphene	40	2–2.5	6–12[b]	6–8	7/8[c,d]
Dihydrocodeine	20	1.6–1.8	3.5–4.5	3–4	4/3[d]
Pentazocine	20	1	3	2–3	1[e]
Tramadol	70[f]	2	6[g]	4–6	2[e]

a. when used in general doses for mild-to-moderate pain
b. increased >50% in the elderly
c. multiple doses; single dose = 1/2–2/3
d. when calculating equivalent doses, can approximate and regard, with codeine, as 1/10 morphine
e. estimated on the basis of potency ratio with morphine
f. multiple doses >90%
g. active metabolite (M1) 7.4h; both figures double in cirrhosis and severe renal failure.

vomiting, if the dose is increased beyond a certain level. The following rules should be observed:

- a weak opioid should be added to a non-opioid, not substituted for one
- if a weak opioid is inadequate when given regularly in an optimal dose, change to morphine (or an alternative strong opioid)
- do not 'kangaroo' from weak opioid to weak opioid.

Codeine is about 1/10 as potent as morphine and, in terms of pain relief, is probably mainly a pro-drug of morphine. *About 10% of the population cannot convert codeine to morphine,*[26] and in consequence obtain little or no analgesia when given it. Codeine is more constipating than other weak opioids, and its use is not generally recommended. Co-proxamol and dihydrocodeine are the weak opioid preparations of choice at many palliative care units in the UK. However, a legitimate option is to skip over step 2 of the WHO ladder and prescribe low-dose morphine instead.

Tramadol

Tramadol forms a bridge between the classic weak and the classic strong opioids and is used at some centres. By injection, it is 1/10 as potent as morphine.[27] By mouth, because of high oral bio-availability, it is more potent and is about 1/5 as potent as morphine.[28]

Tramadol has a dual mechanism of action, partly via opioid receptors and partly (like a tricyclic antidepressant) by blocking the presynaptic re-uptake of 5HT (serotonin) and noradrenaline (norepinephrine). However, unlike tricyclic antidepressants, tramadol does not have antimuscarinic or antidepressant properties. The dual analgesic action is synergistic. Undesirable opioid effects are significantly less than with codeine and morphine.[27] It is less constipating.[29] Because of its non-opioid properties tramadol may be relatively more effective in neuropathic pain than morphine.[30,31]

Tramadol tends to lower seizure threshold. It should be used with caution in patients with epilepsy and in those taking other drugs which lower seizure threshold, e.g. tricyclic antidepressants and SSRIs.

Strong opioid analgesics

Strong opioids exist to be given, not merely to be withheld; their use is dictated by therapeutic need and response, not by brevity of prognosis.

Pain is a physiological antagonist to the central depressant effects of opioids.

Strong opioids do not cause clinically important respiratory depression in patients in pain.[32] Naloxone, a specific opioid antagonist, is rarely needed in palliative care.[33] In contrast to postoperative patients, cancer patients with pain:

- have generally been receiving a weak opioid for some time, i.e. are not opioid naive
- take medication by mouth (slower absorption, lower peak concentration)
- titrate the dose upwards step by step (less likelihood of an excessive dose being given).

The relationship of the therapeutic dose to the lethal dose of a strong opioid (the therapeutic ratio) is greater than commonly supposed. For example, patients who take a double dose of morphine at bedtime are no more likely to die during the night than those who do not.[34]

Tolerance to strong opioids is not a practical problem.[35] Psychological dependence (addiction) does not occur if morphine is used correctly. Physical dependence does not prevent a reduction in the dose of morphine if the patient's pain ameliorates, e.g. as a result of radiotherapy or a nerve block.[36]

Strong opioids are not the panacea for cancer pain; generally they are best administered in conjunction with a non-opioid. However, even combined use does not guarantee success, particularly if the psychosocial dimensions of suffering are ignored.[37]

Oral morphine

Morphine by mouth is the global strong opioid of choice for cancer pain (Box 3.F).[38] It is administered as tablets (e.g. 10mg, 20mg) or in aqueous solutions (e.g. 2mg in 1ml, 20mg in 1ml). An increasing range of m/r preparations is available; tablets, capsules, suspensions. Most are administered b.d., some o.d. There are no generic m/r morphine tablets, but the pharmacokinetic profiles of different proprietary brands are broadly similar.[39]

Morphine is metabolised mainly to morphine-3-glucuronide (M3G) and morphine-6-glucuronide (M6G). M3G is inactive but M6G is more potent than morphine. Both glucuronides cumulate in renal failure. This results in a prolonged duration of action, with a danger of severe sedation and respiratory depression if the dose or frequency of administration is not reduced.

Box 3.F Guidelines for starting a patient on oral morphine

1 Oral morphine is indicated in patients with pain which does not respond to the optimised combined use of a non-opioid and a weak opioid.

2 The starting dose of morphine is calculated to give a greater analgesic effect than the medication already in use:
- if the patient was previously receiving a weak opioid, give 10mg q4h or m/r 20–30mg q12h
- if changing from an alternative strong opioid (e.g. fentanyl, methadone), a much higher dose of morphine may be needed (see p.85)
- if the patient is frail and elderly, a lower dose helps to reduce initial drowsiness, confusion and unsteadiness, e.g. 5mg q4h
- because of cumulation of an active metabolite, a lower and/or less frequent regular dose may be preferable in renal failure, e.g. 5–10mg q6h.

3 If the patient takes two or more p.r.n. doses in 24h, the regular dose should be increased by 30–50% every 2–3 days.

4 Upward titration of the dose of morphine stops when either the pain is relieved or intolerable undesirable effects supervene. In the latter case, it is generally necessary to consider alternative measures. The aim is to have the patient free of pain and mentally alert.

5 *Because of poor absorption, m/r morphine may not be satisfactory in patients troubled by frequent vomiting or those with diarrhoea or an ileostomy. M/r morphine should be used with caution if there is renal impairment.*

6 Supply an anti-emetic in case the patient becomes nauseated, e.g. haloperidol 1.5mg stat & o.n.

7 Prescribe laxatives, e.g. co-danthrusate (see p.112); adjust the dose as necessary. Suppositories and enemas continue to be necessary in about 1/3 of patients. *Constipation may be more difficult to manage than the pain.*

8 Warn all patients about the possibility of initial drowsiness.

9 If swallowing is difficult or there is persistent vomiting, morphine may be given PR by suppository; the dose is the same as PO. Alternatively give 1/2 the oral dose by injection, or 1/3 as diamorphine, preferably by CSCI.

10 For outpatients, write out the drug regimen in detail with times, names of drugs and amount to be taken; arrange for follow-up.

Scheme 1: ordinary (normal-release) morphine tablets or solution
- morphine given q4h regularly 'by the clock' with q1h p.r.n. doses of equal amount
- after 1–2 days, adjust the dose upwards if the patient still has pain or is using two or more p.r.n. doses per day
- continue q4h regularly with q1h p.r.n. doses of equal amount
- increase the regular dose by 30–50% every 2–3 days until there is adequate relief throughout each 4h period

continued

Box 3.F   Continued

- a double dose at bedtime obviates the need to wake the patient for a q4h dose during the night.

Scheme 2: ordinary (normal-release) morphine and modified-release (m/r) morphine
- begin as for Scheme I
- when the q4h dose is stable, replace with m/r morphine q12h, or o.d. if a 24h preparation is prescribed
- the q12h dose will be *three times* the previous q4h dose; an o.d. dose will be *six times* the previous q4h dose, rounded to a convenient number of tablets or capsules
- continue to provide ordinary morphine tablets or solutions for p.r.n. use; give the equivalent of a q4h dose, i.e. 1/6 of the total daily dose.

Scheme 3: m/r morphine and ordinary (normal-release) morphine
- starting dose generally m/r morphine 20–30mg q12h or 40–60mg o.d.
- use ordinary morphine tablets or solution for p.r.n. medication; give about 1/6 of the total daily dose
- increase the dose of m/r morphine by 30–50% every 2–3 days until there is adequate relief around the clock.

Diamorphine

Diamorphine hydrochloride (di-acetylmorphine, heroin) is available for medicinal use only in the UK. It is much more soluble than morphine sulphate/hydrochloride and large amounts can be given in a very small volume. It is used instead of morphine when injections are necessary.

IV diamorphine is twice as potent as IV morphine.[40,41] By this route, its initial effects are mediated by the primary metabolite, mono-acetylmorphine.[42] However, by mouth, diamorphine is virtually a pro-drug for morphine because of its rapid de-acetylation.[43]

When changing from oral diamorphine q4h to m/r morphine, convert 1mg for 1mg and adjust as necessary.

Alternative strong opioids

There are multiple opioid receptor subtypes in the CNS and elsewhere, including the dorsal horn of the spinal cord; μ, κ and δ opioid receptors are all involved in analgesia. Opioids differ from each other in terms of intrinsic activity, receptor site affinity, and non-opioid effects (Table 3.5).[44] These properties can be utilised in patients who are intolerant of morphine by switching to an alternative opioid (Table 3.6).[45] The initial dose of the second opioid depends on the relative potency of the two drugs.

Table 3.5 Alternative strong opioids[44]

| | Opioid receptor affinity | | | Non-opioid properties | Bio-availability | Plasma halflife | Typical duration of action | Preparations available in UK | | | | | Potency ratio with morphine PO[a] |
	Mu	Kappa	Delta					Oral solution	Tablet/capsule	Trans-mucosal	M/r	Injection	
Buprenorphine	pA	Ant	A	None	50–60% SL	3h	6–9h 72h TD	–	–	Tab SL	TD	+	60
Fentanyl	A	–	–	None	–	3h 24h	3–4h 72h TD	–	–	Loz	TD	+	100
Hydromorphone	A	–	–	None	37–62% PO	2.5h	4–5h	–	Cap	–	Cap	+	7.5
Methadone	A	–	A(?)	Inhibits presynaptic serotonin re-uptake, NMDA-receptor-channel blocker	40–100% PO	8–75h	4–6h single dose, 8–12h repeat doses	+	Tab	–	–	+	5–10
Oxycodone	–	A	–	None	60–87% PO	3.5h	4–6h 12h m/r	+	Cap	–	Tab	–	1.5–2

a. these are all debatable but represent safe 'transfer factors'; for discussion, see respective monographs in the *Palliative Care Formulary*.

Key: A = strong agonist; pA = partial agonist; a = weak agonist; Ant = strong antagonist; ant = weak antagonist; – = no activity; m/r = modified-release; Tab = tablet; Cap = capsule; Loz = lozenge; PO = per os, oral; SL = sublingual; TD = transdermal.

Table 3.6 Potential intolerable effects of morphine

Type	Effects	Initial action	Comment
Gastric stasis	Epigastric fullness, flatulence, anorexia, hiccup, persistent nausea	Metoclopramide 10–20mg q4h	If the problem persists, change to an alternative opioid
Sedation	Intolerable persistent sedation	Reduce dose of morphine; consider methylphenidate 10mg o.d.–b.d.	Sedation may be caused by other factors; stimulant rarely appropriate
Cognitive failure	Agitated delirium with hallucinations	Prescribe haloperidol 3–5mg stat & p.r.n.; reduce dose of morphine and, if no improvement, switch to an alternative opioid	Some patients develop intractable delirium with one opioid but not with an alternative opioid
Myoclonus	Multifocal twitching ± jerking of limbs	Prescribe diazepam/midazolam 5mg stat & p.r.n.; reduce dose of morphine but increase again if pain recurs	Unusual with typical oral doses; more common with high-dose IV and spinal morphine
Hyperexcitability	Abdominal muscle spasms, symmetrical jerking of legs; whole-body allodynia, hyperalgesia (manifests as excruciating pain)	Prescribe diazepam/midazolam 5mg stat & p.r.n.; reduce dose of morphine; consider changing to an alternative opioid	A rare syndrome in patients receiving intrathecal or high-dose IV morphine; occasionally seen with typical PO and SC doses

continued

Table 3.6 Continued

Type	Effects	Initial action	Comment
Vestibular stimulation	Movement-induced nausea and vomiting	Prescribe cyclizine or dimenhydrinate or promethazine 25–50mg q8h–q6h	If intractable, try an alternative opioid or levomepromazine (methotrimeprazine)
Pruritus	Whole-body itch with systemic morphine; localised to upper body or face/nose with spinal morphine	Ondansetron 8mg IV stat and 8mg PO b.d. for 3–5 days	This is a central phenomenon and does not respond to H_1-antihistamines; centrally-acting opioid antagonists also relieve the itch but antagonise analgesia[11]
Histamine release	Bronchoconstriction → dyspnoea	Prescribe IV/IM antihistamine (e.g. ch orphenamine 5–10mg) and a bronchodilator; change to a chemically distinct opioid immediately e.g. methadone	Rare

Some patients taking high-dose morphine manifest evidence of hyperexcit-abilility, i.e. myoclonus, allodynia, hyperalgesia. The main causal factor seems to be a cumulation of morphine-3-glucuronide which indirectly antagonises the analgesic effect of morphine, i.e. not via opioid receptors.[46] Thus when switching from morphine, particularly because of hyperexcitability, a lower than expected dose of the alternative opioid is needed.[47,48]

With methadone, the long halflife creates additional difficulties. Single doses of IM morphine and methadone given postoperatively are approximately equipotent.[49] However, when changing from high-dose morphine to metha-done, the effective dose of methadone is likely to be 5–10 times less,[50] and occasionally 20–30 times less (Box 3.G).[51]

Pethidine and dextromoramide have little place in cancer pain management because of short durations of action. However, because of its rapid onset of action, some centres in the UK use dextromoramide SL/PO in patients taking regular morphine for episodic pain or prophylactically before a painful pro-cedure. At other centres oral transmucosal fentanyl citrate (OTFC) is used, despite its cost (over £6 per lozenge). Alternatively, patients can be given an additional dose of morphine, or the procedure timed for 1h after a regular q4h dose of morphine, or 2–3h after m/r morphine.

Fentanyl is a potent μ-opioid receptor agonist.[52] Transdermal patches are avail-able for chronic pain management.[53,54] These deliver 25, 50, 75 or 100mg/h over 3 days. Patients who have not previously taken morphine or another strong opioid should always be started on the lowest dose, i.e. 25mg/h (Box 3.H). After removal of a patch, the elimination plasma halflife is almost 24h,[55] compared with 3–4h after a single IV injection.[56]

Box 3.G   Guidelines for the use of methadone for cancer pain

In addition to being an opioid agonist, methadone is a NMDA-receptor-channel blocker and a presynaptic blocker of serotonin re-uptake. Its plasma halflife varies from about 8–80h.

Indications for use
1 Methadone is used in the following situations:
- severe/intolerable undesirable effects with morphine at any dose, e.g. sedation, hallucinations, dysphoria, delirium, myoclonus, allodynia, hyper-algesia, as an alternative to low-dose spinal morphine or if these effects complicate spinal morphine use
- increasing pain despite increasingly high doses of morphine compounded by intolerable undesirable effects
- neuropathic cancer pain not responding to a typical regimen of a NSAID, morphine, amitriptyline and sodium valproate
- renal failure, where it may be used as the opioid of choice because its metabolism and excretion are unchanged in this circumstance
- only attempt in patients with a prognosis of ⩾10 days.

Therapeutic inequivalence
2 Because methadone is very different from morphine, when switching from high-dose morphine to methadone it is necessary to be aware of opioid *inequivalence*, i.e. the 2 drugs do *not* have a single potency ratio. In practice the 24h dose of methadone is 5–10 times *smaller* than the previous dose of morphine, and sometimes even smaller.

Dose titration
3 For patients in renal failure who have not been on morphine PO, commence on methadone 5–10mg q12h *and* q3h p.r.n. If necessary, titrate the regular dose upwards every 4–6 days.
4 For patients already receiving morphine, use Scheme 1.

Scheme 1 (Morley & Makin, UK)

Stop morphine abruptly; i.e. do *not* reduce progressively over several days.

Prescribe a dose of methadone that is 1/10 of the 24h PO morphine dose *up to a maximum of 30mg.*

Allow the patient to take the prescribed dose *q3h p.r.n.*

On day 6, the amount of methadone taken over the previous 2 days is noted and converted into a regular q12h dose, with provision for a similar or smaller dose q3h p.r.n.

If p.r.n. medication is still needed, increase the dose of methadone by 1/2–1/3 every 4–6 days. [Example: 10mg b.d. → 15mg b.d.; 30mg b.d → 40mg b.d.]

continued

Box 3.G   Continued

5 Because many patients (and staff) have become used to morphine by-the-clock, they are not comfortable with a total p.r.n. regimen. In this case, Scheme 2 may be preferable.

Scheme 2 (Nauck, Germany)

Stop morphine abruptly; i.e. do *not* reduce progressively over several days.

Initially prescribe methadone 5–10mg PO q4h *and* q1h p.r.n. *whatever the dose of morphine.*

After 12–24h, if frequent p.r.n. doses are still needed and the pain is not easing, increase methadone to 10–15mg q4h and q1h p.r.n.

After 72h, reduce regular methadone to q8h *and* q3h p.r.n.

Subsequently, increase the dose of methadone every 4–5 days if still needing multiple p.r.n. doses.

---

6 With both schemes, morphine (or other opioid) is stopped abruptly.

7 *Particularly over the first 48h, the patient may experience significant pain but if the switch is successful, the pain steadily diminishes and p.r.n. doses of methadone similarly.*
   A failed conversion is obvious: pain remains unrelieved and the intervals between doses do not lengthen, or the patient experiences undue undesirable effects without adequate analgesia.

8 When the b.d. dose has been determined, methadone can continue to be used as rescue medication for breakthrough pain.

SC methadone
9 CSCI infusion of methadone causes a skin reaction; this is reduced if:
   - a more dilute solution is used, e.g. a 20–30ml syringe
   - the syringe is changed b.d.
   - the site is changed every day.

10 An arbitrary SC methadone dose of 1/20 the previous dose of SC morphine is a safe dose. In patients on morphine ≤1g/24h, it is generally safe to give 1/10.
   When converting from PO methadone to SC methadone, give 1/2 the PO dose.

11 Additional rescue doses of methadone can be given for breakthrough pain, using 1/5–1/6 of the 24h infusion dose q3h p.r.n.

12 If necessary, p.r.n. doses of morphine (or other previously used strong opioid) can be given q1h, based on previous morphine requirements.

13 The dose of methadone should be increased if p.r.n. doses are still needed after several days.

Box 3.H   Guidelines for the use of transdermal fentanyl patches

1 Transdermal (TD) fentanyl is an alternative strong opioid which can be used in place of both PO morphine and CSCI morphine/diamorphine in the management of cancer pain.

2 Indications for using TD fentanyl include:
- intolerable undesirable effects with morphine, e.g. nausea and vomiting, constipation, hallucinations
- renal failure (no active metabolite)
- dysphagia
- 'tablet phobia' or poor compliance with oral medication.

3 TD fentanyl is *contra-indicated* in patients who need rapid titration of their medication for severe uncontrolled pain.
Pain not relieved by morphine will *not* be relieved by fentanyl. If in doubt, seek specialist advice before prescribing TD fentanyl.

4 TD fentanyl patches are available in 4 strengths: 25, 50, 75, 100microgram/h *for 3 days*:
- patients with inadequate relief from codeine, dextropropoxyphene or dihydrocodeine ⩾240mg/day should start on 25microgram/h
- patients on oral morphine: *divide 24h dose in mg by 3* and choose nearest patch strength in microgram/h
- patients on CSCI diamorphine: choose nearest patch strength in microgram/h to mg/24h of diamorphine.
Note: the latter two doses are higher than the manufacturer's recommendations.

5 An alternative method of deciding the initial patch strength is to use a potency ratio of 100 (as in Germany) and to round down to the nearest convenient patch size.
[Example: morphine daily dose 120mg ÷ 100 = fentanyl daily dose 1.2mg, i.e. patch strength 50microgram/h.]

6 Apply the patch to *dry, non-inflamed, non-irradiated, hairless skin* on the upper arm or trunk; body hair may be clipped but not shaved. May need micropore to ensure adherence.

7 Systemic analgesic concentrations are generally reached within 12h; so if converting from:
- 4-hourly oral morphine, give regular doses for the first 12h after applying the patch
- 12-hourly m/r morphine, apply the patch and the final m/r dose at the same time
- 24-hourly m/r morphine, apply the patch 12h after the final m/r dose
- a syringe driver, continue the syringe driver for about 12h after applying the patch.

8 Steady-state plasma concentrations of fentanyl are achieved after 36–48h; the patient should use p.r.n. doses liberally during the first 3 days, particularly during the first 24h. Rescue doses should be approximately half the fentanyl patch strength given as normal-release morphine in mg. [Example: with fentanyl 50microgram/h, use morphine 20–30mg p.r.n.]

continued

Box 3.H   Continued

9 After 48h, if a patient continues to need 2 or more rescue doses of morphine a day, the patch strength should be increased by 25microgram/h. When using the manufacturer's recommended starting doses, about 50% of patients need to increase the patch strength after the first 3 days.

10 About 10% of patients experience opioid withdrawal symptoms when changed from morphine to TD fentanyl. These manifest with symptoms like gastric flu and last for a few days; p.r.n. doses of morphine can be used to relieve troublesome symptoms.

11 Fentanyl is less constipating than morphine; halve the dose of laxatives when starting fentanyl and titrate according to need. Some patients develop diarrhoea; if troublesome, use rescue doses of morphine to control it, and completely stop laxatives.

12 Fentanyl probably causes less nausea and vomiting than morphine but, if necessary, prescribe haloperidol 1.5mg stat and o.n.

13 In febrile patients, the rate of absorption of fentanyl increases, and occasionally causes toxicity, principally drowsiness. Absorption may also be enhanced by an external heat source over the patch, e.g. electric blanket or hot-water bottle; patients should be warned about this. Patients may shower with a patch but should not soak in a hot bath.

14 Remove patches after 72h; change the position of the new patches so as to rest the underlying skin for 3–6 days.

15 A reservoir of fentanyl cumulates in the skin under the patch, and significant blood levels persist for 24h, sometimes more, after removing the patch. This only matters, of course, if transdermal fentanyl is discontinued.

16 In moribund patients, continue TD fentanyl and give additional diamorphine p.r.n. Rescue doses of SC diamorphine can be based on the 'rule of 5', i.e. divide the patch strength by 5 and give as mg of diamorphine. [Example: with fentanyl 100microgram/h, use diamorphine 20mg p.r.n.] If ⩾2 p.r.n. doses are required/24h, give diamorphine by CSCI, starting with a dose equal to the sum of the p.r.n. doses over the preceding 24h. The p.r.n. dose may need to be adjusted taking into account the total opioid dose (i.e. fentanyl TD and diamorphine CSCI).

17 TD fentanyl is unsatisfactory in <5% of patients, generally because of failure to remain adherent or allergy to the silicone adhesive.

18 Used patches still contain fentanyl; after removal, fold the patch with the adhesive side inwards and discard in a sharps container (hospital) or dustbin (home); wash hands. Ultimately any unused patches should be returned to a pharmacy.

Adjuvant analgesics

Adjuvant analgesics are a miscellaneous group of drugs which relieve pain in specific circumstances (Table 3.7).[57] Although sometimes used alone, they are generally 'add-on' drugs supplementing the impact of an NSAID and an opioid (Figure 3.8).

It is important to establish a straightforward practical scheme for neuropathic pain management, selecting only one or two drugs from each category of agents (Figure 3.9)[58,59] About 90% of patients with nerve injury pain respond well to the systematic use of non-opioids, opioids and adjuvant analgesics.[6] The remainder require spinal analgesia (e.g. morphine + bupivacaine ± clonidine) or a neurolytic procedure to obtain adequate relief. Some patients derive benefit from other non-drug measures, e.g. transcutaneous electrical nerve stimulation (TENS).

Generally, with neuropathic pain the crucial first step is to help the patient obtain a good night's sleep. The second is to reduce pain intensity and allodynia to a bearable level during the day. Initially there may be marked diurnal variation in relief, with more prolonged periods with less or no pain rather than a decrease in worst pain intensity around the clock.

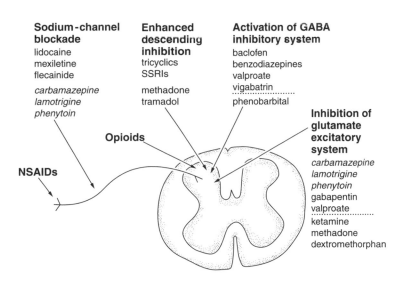

Figure 3.8 Primary site of action of analgesics and adjuvant analgesics on peripheral nerves and the dorsal horn of the spinal cord. Drugs in italics act both peripherally and centrally. Drugs below the dotted lines are channel blockers at their respective receptor-channel complex.

Table 3.7　Adjuvant analgesics[a]

Class	Main indications	Mechanism(s) of action	Examples	Typical regimen	Undesirable effects
Corticosteroids	Nerve compression Spinal cord compression	Reduce peri-tumour oedema	Prednisolone Dexamethasone	15–30mg o.m. 8–16mg o.m.	Include hyperglycaemia, anxiety, steroid psychosis, myopathy
Antidepressants	Nerve injury pain	Potentiation of two spinal descending inhibitory pathways	Amitriptyline Imipramine	25–100mg o.n	Antimuscarinic effects, drowsiness, postural hypotension (particularly amitriptyline)
Anti-epileptics	Nerve injury pain	Potentiation of GABA inhibitory and glutamate excitatory mechanisms in dorsal horn	Sodium valproate	400–1000mg o.n.	Drowsiness
		Selective calcium-channel blockade	Gabapentin	100–300mg t.d.s.	Drowsiness
NMDA-receptor-channel blockers	Pain poorly responsive to analgesic	Block channel in NMDA-type glutamate-receptor-channel	Methadone Ketamine	10–60mg b.d. 100–500mg/24h SC 10–20mg q6h PO	Drowsiness (methadone), dysphoria (ketamine)
Antispasmodics	Bowel colic	Relax intestinal smooth muscle	Hyoscine butylbromide Glycopyrronium	60–160mg/24h SC 600–1200 microgram/24h SC	Peripheral antimuscarinic effects
Muscle relaxants	Muscle spasm	Relax somatic muscle	Diazepam Baclofen	5–10mg o.n. 10mg t.d.s.	Drowsiness, ataxia
Bisphosphonates[60]	Intractable metastatic bone pain	Block osteoclast activity	Pamidronate Zoledronic acid	90mg IV every 4 weeks 4mg IV every 4-8 weeks	Pyrexia, flu-like malaise for 1–2 days (uncommon with zoledronic acid)

a.　choice of drug and dose varies widely, particularly for adjuvant analgesics for neuropathic pain.

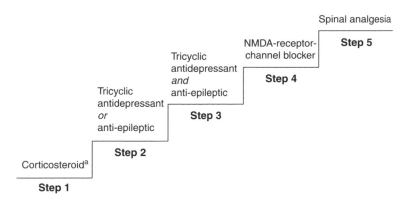

Figure 3.9 Adjuvant analgesics for neuropathic pain. If caused by cancer, use only if the pain does not respond to the combined use of a NSAID and a strong opioid.
a. trial of a corticosteroid is important when neuropathic pain is associated with limb weakness.

The patient should be warned that major benefit often takes a week or more to manifest, although improvement in sleep should occur immediately. Undesirable drug effects tend to be the limiting therapeutic factor.

To avoid excessive drowsiness with psychotropic drugs, dose escalation generally should be relatively slow, e.g. a dose increase no more than twice weekly. However, with a corticosteroid, it is generally best to start with a high dose and then reduce to a satisfactory maintenance level.

NMDA-receptor-channel blockers

NMDA-receptor-channel blockers are used most commonly when neuropathic pain does not respond well to standard analgesics together with an antidepressant and an anti-epileptic. They include:

- methadone (see p.85)[61,62]
- ketamine[63-65]
- amantidine, e.g. 100mg PO b.d.[66,67]

Ketamine

Ketamine is an anaesthetic induction agent. Its plasma halflife is about 3h, and it has an active metabolite, norketamine, with a halflife of 12h.[68] PO doses of ketamine yield lower plasma ketamine concentrations but higher norketamine ones; in chronic use, norketamine may be the main analgesic agent. Its use IV, SC or PO as an analgesic is beyond the manufacturer's licence.[69]

Dose recommendations vary considerably but ketamine is often started in a low dose PO, or even SL.[70] Ketamine is unusual in that the PO doses are often much lower than those given SC. Psychotomimetic effects are common and are treated with haloperidol, diazepam or midazolam.[71] Ketamine has been used IV with fentanyl and midazolam to control intractable pain and agitation.[72,73]

Antispasmodics

Antispasmodics is the term given to antimuscarinic drugs used to relieve visceral distension pain and colic. In advanced cancer, there is little place for 'weak' antispasmodics such as dicycloverine (dicyclomine) and mebeverine. In the UK, hyoscine *butylbromide* is widely regarded as the antispasmodic of choice. This is given by SC injection, i.e. 20mg stat and p.r.n., and 40–160mg by CSCI. In the USA, where hyoscine *butylbromide* is not available, SC glycopyrronium can be substituted, e.g. 200–400microgram stat and p.r.n., and 600–1200microgram/24h by CSCI.

Muscle relaxants

For painful muscle spasm (cramp) and myofascial pain, the correct approach is:

- explanation
- physical therapy (local heat and massage)
- diazepam and relaxation therapy
- injection of the trigger points with local anaesthetic and a corticosteroid (e.g. bupivacaine 0.5% and depot methylprednisolone 80mg).

However severe, morphine is not indicated for the relief of cramp and trigger point pains because it is ineffective.

Bisphosphonates

Bisphosphonates are osteoclast inhibitors and are used to relieve metastatic bone pain which persists despite analgesics and radiotherapy ± orthopaedic surgery. Published data relate mainly to breast cancer and myeloma; benefit is also seen with other cancers. About 50% of patients benefit, typically in 7–14 days, and this may last for 2–3 months. Benefit may be seen only after a second treatment but, if there is no response after two treatments, nothing is gained by further use.[60] In those who respond, continue to treat p.r.n. for as long as there is benefit.

Alternative routes of administration

Not all patients are able to swallow tablets or capsules and those experiencing nausea and vomiting may not be able to retain them. A range of alternative routes is available. In practice, choice is largely determined by commercial availability (Figure 3.10).

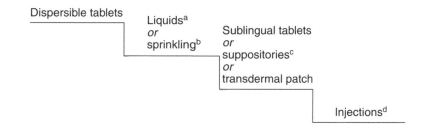

Figure 3.10 Alternative routes of administration.
a. solutions or suspensions
b. on semi-solid food
c. can use m/r tablets
d. CSCI preferable.

'Sprinkling' refers to the practice of emptying the contents of a m/r morphine capsule onto a teaspoon of semi-solid food immediately before swallowing, e.g. apple sauce, puree, jam, yoghurt, ice-cream. Although sachets of m/r morphine granules are available for use as a suspension, they are much more expensive.

Various buccal and sublingual tablets are available, e.g. piroxicam and buprenorphine. Lingual piroxicam (Feldene Melt) is in fact a soluble oral preparation, i.e. the dissolved tablet still has to be swallowed. On the other hand, SL buprenorphine is absorbed locally, and swallowing it results in a major loss of efficacy because of first-pass hepatic metabolism. Oral trans-mucosal fentanyl citrate (OTFC) is used at some centres for breakthrough pain.[74]

Morphine is slowly absorbed through the buccal mucosa,[74] and it can be used by this route in moribund patients being cared for at home. M/r morphine suppositories for o.d. or b.d. use makes PR administration more practical.[75] Although not licensed for this route, m/r morphine tablets have been used PR to provide emergency analgesia in moribund patients.

Continuous SC infusions (CSCI)

Battery-driven portable syringe drivers (Figure 3.12) are a convenient method for administering many drugs by CSCI to patients with severe nausea and vomiting, or who cannot swallow medication for various reasons.[69] The advantages of CSCI infusion include:

- better control of nausea and vomiting (guarantees drug absorption)
- constant analgesia (no peaks or troughs)
- generally reloaded once in 24h (saves nurses' time)
- comfort and confidence (minimal number of injections)
- does not limit mobility (lightweight and compact).

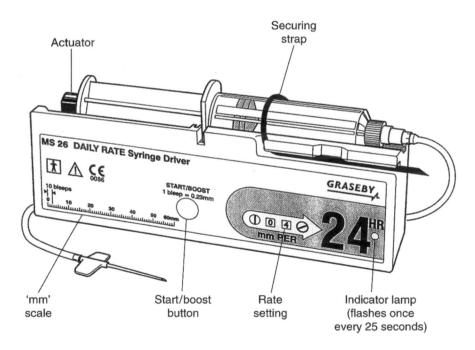

Figure 3.11 The SIMS Graseby MS26.

The most common choices for infusion are:

- upper chest (intercostal plane)
- upper arm (outer aspect)
- abdomen
- thighs.

If the infusion causes painful local inflammation, consider the following options:

- change the needle site prophylactically, e.g. daily
- reduce the quantity of the irritant drug or increase the volume infused
- change to an alternative drug, e.g. cyclizine to hyoscine butylbromide
- give the irritant drug IM or PR
- use a plastic cannula instead of a metal needle
- give a stat injection of hydrocortisone sodium succinate 25–50mg through the butterfly needle and add the same amount to the syringe (not used by the authors)
- give a stat injection of hyaluronidase 1500IU through the butterfly needle and add the same amount to the syringe (not used by the authors).

More information about CSCI, can be found in the *Palliative Care Formulary*[76] or at www.palliativedrugs.com. In patients with venous access, e.g. a Hickman line, the IV route is an obvious alternative but CSCI is generally preferable.

Topical morphine

Nociceptive afferent nerve fibres contain peripheral opioid receptors which are silent except in the presence of local inflammation.[77,78] This property is exploited in joint surgery where morphine is given intra-articularly at the end of the operation.[79] Topical morphine has also been used successfully to relieve otherwise intractable pain associated with cutaneous ulceration, often sacral decubitus.[80–82] Generally it is given as a 0.1% (1mg/ml) gel, in Intrasite. A higher dose may be necessary, e.g. 0.3–0.5%, in other situations:

- oral mucositis
- vaginal inflammation associated with a fistula
- rectal ulceration.[81]

The amount of gel applied varies according to the size and the site of the ulcer but is typically 5–10ml applied b.d.–t.d.s. The topical morphine is kept in place with:

- a non-absorbable pad or dressing, e.g. Opsite
- gauze coated with petroleum jelly.

Spinal morphine

If given epidurally (ED) or intrathecally (IT), a much lower dose of morphine has a much greater analgesic effect because of the proximity to the opioid receptors in the dorsal horn of the spinal cord. The ED dose is about 1/10 and the IT dose 1/100 of the dose of PO morphine. Undesirable effects are correspondingly reduced. In the UK, 5% of cancer patients needing morphine receive it spinally.

The main indications for spinal morphine are:

- intractable pain despite the appropriate combined use of standard and adjuvant analgesics
- intolerable undesirable effects with systemic opioids.

To increase the effect of spinal analgesia in neuropathic pain, morphine is often combined with bupivacaine, and sometimes clonidine.

References

1 Gordon L (1997) *If You Really Loved Me.* Science and Behaviour Books, Palo Alto.
2 IASP Task Force on Taxonomy (1994) *Classification of Chronic Pain.* IASP Press, Seattle.
3 Grond S *et al.* (1996) Assessment of cancer pain: a prospective evaluation in 2266 cancer patients referred to a pain service. *Pain.* **64:** 107–114.
4 IASP (1986) Subcommittee on Taxonomy. Classification of chronic pain. *Pain.* **Suppl 3:** 1–225.
5 Grond S *et al.* (1999) Assessment and treatment of neuropathic cancer pain following WHO guidelines. *Pain.* **79:** 15–20.
6 Twycross R and Wilcock A (2001) *Symptom Management in Advanced Cancer* (3e). Radcliffe Medical Press, Oxford.
7 Geisslinger G and Yaksh T (2000) Spinal actions of cyclooxygenase isozyme inhibitors. In: M Devor *et al.* (eds) *Proceedings of the 9th World Congress on Pain. Progress in Pain Research and Management.* Volume 16. IASP Press, Seattle, pp 771–785.
8 Stein C (1993) Peripheral mechanisms of opioid analgesia. *Anesthesia and Analgesia.* **76:** 182–191.
9 World Health Organization (1986) *Cancer Pain Relief.* WHO, Geneva.
10 Flower RJ and Vane JR (1972) Inhibition of prostaglandin synthetase in brain explains the anti-pyretic activity of paracetamol. *Nature.* **240:** 410–411.
11 Twycross R *et al.* (2002) *Palliative Care Formulary* (2e). Radcliffe Medical Press, Abingdon, Oxon, pp 136–139.
12 Moore U *et al.* (1992) The efficacy of locally applied aspirin and acetaminophen in postoperative pain after third molar surgery. *Clinical Pharmacology and Therapeutics.* **52:** 292–296.
13 Settipane R *et al.* (1995) Prevalence of cross-sensitivity with acetaminophen in aspirin-sensitive asthmatic subjects. *Journal of Allergy and Clinical Immunology.* **96:** 480–485.
14 Dellemijn P *et al.* (1994) Medical therapy of malignant nerve pain. A randomised double-blind explanatory trial with naproxen versus slow-release morphine. *European Journal of Cancer.* **30A:** 1244–1250.
15 McCormack K and Brune K (1991) Dissociation between the antinociceptive and anti-inflammatory effects of the nonsteroidal anti-inflammatory drugs: a survey of their analgesic efficacy. *Drugs.* **41:** 533–547.
16 Simon L *et al.* (2000) Anti-inflammatory and upper gastrointestinal effects of celecoxib in rheumatoid arthritis. *Journal of the American Medical Association.* **282:** 1921–1928.
17 Langman M *et al.* (1999) Adverse upper gastrointestinal effects of rofecoxib compared with NSAIDs. *Journal of the American Medical Association.* **282:** 1929–1933.

18 Somasundaran S et al. (1995) The biochemical basis of nonsteroidal anti-inflammatory drug-induced damage to the gastrointestinal tract: a review and a hypothesis. *Scandinavian Journal of Gastroenterology.* **30:** 289–299.

19 Bennett A (2000) The importance of COX-2 inhibition for aspirin induced asthma. *Thorax.* **55:** S54–S56.

20 Stockley I (1999) Hypoglycaemic agents and salicylates. In: I Stockley (ed) *Textbook of Drug Interactions* (5e). Pharmaceutical Press, London, pp 528–529.

21 Todd P and Sorkin E (1988) Diclofenac sodium: a reappraisal of its pharmacodynamic and pharmacokinetic properties, and therapeutic efficacy. *Drugs.* **35:** 244–285.

22 Cullen L et al. (1997) Selective suppression of cyclooxygenase-2 during chronic administration of nimesulide in man. *Presented at the Fourth International Congress on essential fatty acids and eicosanoids.* Edinburgh.

23 Clemett D and Goa K (2000) Celecoxib: a review of its use in osteoarthritis, rheumatoid arthritis and acute pain. *Drugs.* **59:** 957–980.

24 Guth B et al. (1996) Therapeutic doses of meloxicam do not inhibit platelet aggregation in man. *Rheumatology in Europe.* **25:** Abstract 443.

25 van Hecken A et al. (2000) Comparative inhibitory activity of rofecoxib, meloxicam, diclofenac, ibuprofen and naproxen on COX-2 versus COX-1 in healthy volunteers. *Journal of Clinical Pharmacology.* **40:** 1109–1120.

26 Hanks G and Cherry N (1997) Opioid analgesic therapy. In: D Doyle et al. (eds) *Oxford Textbook of Palliative Medicine.* Oxford University Press, Oxford, pp 331–355.

27 Vickers M et al. (1992) Tramadol: pain relief by an opioid without depression of respiration. *Anaesthesia.* **47:** 291–296.

28 Wilder-Smith C et al. (1994) Oral tramadol and morphine for strong cancer-related pain. *Annals of Oncology.* **5:** 141–146.

29 Wilder-Smith C and Bettiga A (1997) The analgesic tramadol has minimal effect on gastro-intestinal motor function. *British Journal of Clinical Pharmacology.* **43:** 71–75.

30 Sindrup S and Jensen T (1999) Efficacy of pharmacological treatments of neuropathic pain: an update and effect related to mechanism of drug action. *Pain.* **83:** 389–400.

31 Sindrup S et al. (1999) Tramadol relieves pain and allodynia in polyneuropathy: a randomised, double-blind, controlled trial. *Pain.* **83:** 85–90.

32 Borgbjerg FM et al. (1996) Experimental pain stimulates respiration and attenuates morphine-induced respiratory depression: a controlled study in human volunteers. *Pain.* **64:** 123–128.

33 Twycross R et al. (2002) *Palliative Care Formulary* (2e). Radcliffe Medical Press, Oxford, pp 199–201.

34 Regnard CFB and Badger C (1987) Opioids, sleep and the time of death. *Palliative Medicine.* **1:** 107–110.

35 Collin E et al. (1993) Is disease progression the major factor in morphine 'tolerance' in cancer pain treatment? *Pain.* **55:** 319–326.

36 Twycross RG and Wald SJ (1976) Longterm use of diamorphine in advanced cancer. In: JJ Bonica and D Albe-Fessard (eds) *Advances in Pain Research and Therapy.* Vol 1. Raven Press, New York, pp 653–661.

37 Hanks G et al. (2001) Morphine and alternative opioids in cancer pain: the EAPC recommendations. *British Journal of Cancer.* **84:** 587–593.

38 World Health Organization (1996) *Cancer Pain Relief: with a guide to opioid availability* (2e). WHO, Geneva.

39 Collins S et al. (1998) Peak plasma concentrations after oral morphine: a systematic review. *Journal of Pain and Symptom Management.* **16:** 388–402.

40 Smith GM et al. (1962) Subjective effects of heroin and morphine in normal subjects. *Journal of Pharmacology and Experimental Therapeutics.* **136:** 47–52.

41 Loan WB et al. (1969) Studies of drugs given before anaesthesia. XVII. The natural and semi-synthetic opiates. *British Journal of Anaesthesiology.* **41:** 57–63.

42 Wright CI and Barbour FA (1935) The respiratory effects of morphine, codeine and related substances. *Journal of Pharmacology and Experimental Therapeutics.* **54:** 25–33.

43 Twycross RG (1977) Choice of strong analgesic in terminal cancer: diamorphine or morphine? *Pain.* **3:** 93–104.

44 Twycross R *et al.* (2002) *Palliative Care Formulary* (2e). Radcliffe Medical Press, Oxford, pp 168–198.

45 Ashby M *et al.* (1999) Opioid substitution to reduce adverse effects in cancer pain management. *Medical Journal of Australia.* **170:** 68–71.

46 Smith M (2000) Neuroexcitatory effects of morphine and hydromorphone: evidence implicating the 3-glucuronide metabolites. *Clinical and Experimental Pharmacology and Physiology.* **27:** 524–528.

47 Bruera E *et al.* (1996) Opioid rotation in patients with cancer pain. *Cancer.* **78:** 852–857.

48 Lawlor P *et al.* (1998) Dose ratio between morphine and methadone in patients with cancer pain. *Cancer.* **82:** 1167–1173.

49 Beaver WT *et al.* (1967) A clinical comparison of the analgesic effects of methadone and morphine administered intramuscularly, and of orally and parenterally administered methadone. *Clinical Pharmacology and Therapeutics.* **8:** 415–426.

50 Gagnon B and Bruera E (1999) Differences in the ratios of morphine to methadone in patients with neuropathic pain versus non-neuropathic pain. *Journal of Pain and Symptom Management.* **18:** 120–125.

51 Blackburn D *et al.* (2002) Methadone: an alternative conversion regime. *European Journal of Palliative Care.* **9:** 93–96.

52 Twycross R *et al.* (2002) *Palliative Care Formulary* (2e). Radcliffe Medical Press, Oxford, pp 184–190.

53 Gourlay GK *et al.* (1989) The transdermal administration of fentanyl in the treatment of post-operative pain: pharmacokinetics and pharmacodynamic effects. *Pain.* **37:** 193–202.

54 Ahmedzai S and Brooks D (1997) Transdermal fentanyl versus sustained-release oral morphine in cancer pain: preference, efficacy and quality of life. *Journal of Pain and Symptom Management.* **13:** 254–261.

55 Portenoy RK *et al.* (1993) Transdermal fentanyl for cancer pain. *Anesthesiology.* **78:** 36–43.

56 Hammack JE and Loprinzi CL (1994) Use of orally administered opioids for cancer-related pain. *Mayo Clinic Proceedings.* **69:** 384–390.

57 Twycross R *et al.* (2002) *Palliative Care Formulary* (2e). Radcliffe Medical Press, Oxford, pp 131–136.

58 Chabal C *et al.* (1992) The use of oral mexiletine for the treatment of pain after peripheral nerve injury. *Anaesthesiology.* **76:** 513–517.

59 Chong S *et al.* (1997) Pilot study evaluating local anesthetics administered systemically for treatment of pain in patients with advanced cancer. *Journal of Pain and Symptom Management.* **13:** 112–117.

60 Mannix K *et al.* (2000) Using bisphosphonates to control the pain of bone metastases: evidence-based guidelines for palliative care. *Palliative Medicine.* **14:** 455–461.

61 Gannon C (1997) The use of methadone in the care of the dying. *European Journal of Palliative Care.* **4:** 152–158.

62 Morley J and Makin M (1998) The use of methadone in cancer pain poorly responsive to other opioids. *Pain Reviews.* **5:** 51–58.

63 Enarson M *et al.* (1999) Clinical experience with oral ketamine. *Journal of Pain and Symptom Management.* **17:** 384–386.

64 Fine P (1999) Low-dose ketamine in the management of opioid nonresponsive terminal cancer. *Journal of Pain and Symptom Management.* **17:** 296–300.

65 Finlay I (1999) Ketamine and its role in cancer pain. *Pain Reviews.* **6:** 303–313.

66 Kornhuber J *et al.* (1995) Therapeutic brain concentration of the NMDA receptor antagonist amantadine. *Neuropharmacology.* **34:** 713–721.

67 Pud D *et al.* (1998) The NMDA receptor antagonist amantadine reduces surgical neuropathic pain in cancer patients: a double blind, randomized, placebo controlled trial. *Pain.* **75:** 349–354.

68 Domino E *et al.* (1984) Ketamine kinetics in unmedicated and diazepam premedicated subjects. *Clinical Pharmacology and Therapeutics.* **36:** 645–653.

69 Twycross R *et al.* (2002) *Palliative Care Formulary* (2e). Radcliffe Medical Press, Oxford.

70 Batchelor G (1999) Ketamine in neuropathic pain. *The Pain Society Newsletter.* **1:** 19.

71 Fisher K and Hagen N (1999) Analgesic effect of oral ketamine in chronic neuropathic pain of spinal origin: a case report. *Journal of Pain and Symptom Management.* **18:** 61–66.

72 Berger J *et al.* (2000) Ketamine-fentanyl-midazolam infusion for the control of symptoms in terminal life care. *American Journal of Hospice and Palliative Care.* **17:** 127–132.

73 Enck R (2000) A ketamine, fentanyl, and midazolam infusion for uncontrolled terminal pain and agitation. *American Journal of Hospice and Palliative Care.* **17:** 76–77.

74 Coluzzi P (1998) Sublingual morphine: efficacy reviewed. *Journal of Pain and Symptom Management.* **16:** 184–192.

75 Bruera E *et al.* (1999) Twice-daily versus once-daily morphine sulphate controlled-release suppositories for the treatment of cancer pain. *Supportive Care in Cancer.* **7:** 280–283.

76 Twycross R *et al.* (2002) *Palliative Care Formulary* (2e). Radcliffe Medical Press, Oxford, pp 297–303.

77 Krajnik M and Zylicz Z (1997) Topical opioids – fact or fiction? *Progress in Palliative Care.* **5:** 101–106.

78 Krajnik M *et al.* (1998) Opioids affect inflammation and the immune system. *Pain Reviews.* **5:** 147–154.

79 Likar R *et al.* (1999) Dose-dependency of intra-articular morphine analgesia. *British Journal of Anaesthesia.* **83:** 241–244.

80 Back NI and Finlay I (1995) Analgesic effect of topical opioids on painful skin ulcers. *Journal of Pain and Symptom Management.* **10:** 493.

81 Krajnik M *et al.* (1999) Potential uses of topical opioids in palliative care – report of 6 cases. *Pain.* **80:** 121–125.

82 Twillman R *et al.* (1999) Treatment of painful skin ulcers with topical opioids. *Journal of Pain and Symptom Management.* **17:** 288–292.

PART FOUR

Symptom management II

Alimentary symptoms · Respiratory symptoms
Urinary symptoms · Other symptoms
Secondary mental disorders

Alimentary symptoms

Anorexia

Anorexia (poor appetite) is common in advanced cancer. Anorexia may be primary as in the cachexia-anorexia syndrome (*see* p.107) or secondary to one or more other conditions (Table 4.1).

Table 4.1   Causes of poor appetite in advanced cancer

Causes	*Management possibilities*
Unappetising food	Choice of food by patient
Too much food provided	Small meals
Altered taste	Adjust diet to counter taste changes
Dyspepsia	Antacid, antiflatulent, prokinetic drug
Nausea and vomiting	Anti-emetics
Early satiety ⎫ Fatigue ⎭	'Small and often', snacks rather than meals
Gastric stasis	Prokinetic drug
Constipation	Laxatives
Sore mouth	Mouth care
Pain	Analgesics
Malodour	Treatment of malodour
Biochemical	
hypercalcaemia	Correction of hypercalcaemia
hyponatraemia	Demeclocycline 300mg b.d.–q.d.s. if caused by SIADH
uraemia	Anti-emetic
Secondary to treatment	
drugs	Modify drug regimen
radiotherapy ⎫ chemotherapy ⎭	Anti-emetics
Disease process	Appetite stimulant
Anxiety	Anxiolytic
Depression	Antidepressant

Although anorexia and early satiety often co-exist, early satiety also occurs without anorexia ('I look forward to my meals but, then, after a few mouthfuls I feel full up and can't eat any more'). Causes of early satiety without anorexia include:

- a small stomach (postgastrectomy)
- hepatomegaly
- gross ascites.

Management

Whose problem is it? The patient's or the family's?

Helping the patient and family accept and adjust to the reduced appetite is often the focus of management:

- listen to the family's fears
- explain to the family that
    in the circumstances it is normal to be satisfied with less food
    they can assist a fickle appetite by providing food when the patient is hungry (a microwave oven helps with this)
- a small helping looks better on a smaller plate
- offer specific dietary advice, particularly with early satiety
- discourage the 'he must eat or he'll die' syndrome by emphasising that a balanced diet is unnecessary at this stage in the illness
    'Just give him a little of what he fancies'
    'I shall be happy even if he just takes fluids'
- recognise the 'food as love' and 'feeding him is my job' syndromes and use them as an opportunity to discuss the progressive impact of the illness with the spouse/partner
- remember that eating is a social habit; people generally eat better at a table and when dressed.

Appetite stimulants are appropriate in only a minority of anorexic patients. If used, they should be closely monitored and stopped if no benefit is perceived after 1–2 weeks:

- corticosteroid, e.g. prednisolone 15–30mg o.m. or dexamethasone 2–4mg o.m.; useful in about 50% of patients but the effect generally lasts for only a few weeks[1,2]
- progestogen, e.g. megesterol 160–800mg o.m.; the effect may last for months and is often associated with weight gain.[3,4]

Appetite stimulants are contra-indicated for early satiety without concurrent anorexia.

Cachexia

Cachexia (marked weight loss and muscle wasting) is often associated with anorexia as the cachexia-anorexia syndrome.

Causes

Cachexia occurs in over 50% of patients with advanced cancer.[5] The incidence is highest in gastro-intestinal and lung cancers. Unlike starvation where muscle mass is largely preserved, in cachexia there is a marked reduction in both muscle mass and body fat.[6] The loss of muscle relates to increased levels of proteolysis-inducing factor.[7]

Cachexia is not correlated with food intake or the stage of the tumour. It may antedate the clinical diagnosis and can occur with a small primary neoplasm.[8] The cachexia-anorexia syndrome is a paraneoplastic phenomenon which may be exacerbated by various factors (Box 4.A). Cytokine production suggests a chronic inflammatory component, which explains the beneficial effect of ibuprofen in some patients.[9,10]

Box 4.A Causes of cachexia in advanced cancer

Paraneoplastic
Cytokines produced by host cells and tumour, e.g.
  tumour necrosis factor
  interleukin-6
  interleukin-1
Proteolysis-inducing factor →
abnormal metabolism of
  protein
  carbohydrate
Altered fat metabolism
Increased metabolic rate → increased energy expenditure
Nitrogen trap by the tumour

Concurrent
Anorexia → deficient food intake
Vomiting
Diarrhoea
Malabsorption
Bowel obstruction
Debilitating effect of treatment
  surgery
  radiotherapy
  chemotherapy
Ulceration ⎫ excessive loss
Haemorrhage ⎭ of body protein

Clinical features

The principal features of the cachexia-anorexia syndrome are:

● marked weight loss
● anorexia

- weakness
- fatigue.

Associated physical features include:

- altered taste sensation
- loose dentures causing pain and difficulty with eating
- pallor (anaemia)
- oedema (hypo-albuminaemia)
- pressure sores.

Psychosocial ramifications extend to:

- ill-fitting clothes which increase the sense of loss and displacement
- altered appearance which engenders fear and isolation
- difficulties in social and family relationships.

Management

Because of abnormal metabolism, aggressive dietary supplementation via a nasogastric tube or IV hyperalimentation is of little value in cachexia in advanced cancer.[11] Even so, dietary advice is important, particularly if there are associated changes in taste sensation. Some patients benefit psychologically from powdered or liquid nutritional supplements, and a few gain weight.[12]

Efforts should be directed towards ameliorating the social consequences and physical complications:

- do not weigh the patient routinely
- educate the patient and family about the risk of decubitus ulcers and the importance of skin care
- if affordable, buy new clothes to enhance self-esteem
- reline dentures to improve chewing and facial appearance; as a temporary measure, this can be done at the bedside and lasts about 3 months
- supply equipment to help maintain personal independence, e.g. raised toilet seat, commode, walking frame, wheelchair.

A trial of therapy with a corticosteroid,[13] followed possibly by a progestogen, is sometimes worthwhile.[3,14,15] However, progestogens are expensive and should be used selectively. The effect of progestogens may be enhanced by the concurrent use of ibuprofen 1200mg/day or other NSAID.[16]

Constipation

Constipation (difficulty in defaecation) is common in advanced cancer. Diminished food and fibre intake, lack of exercise and drugs are all contributory. Because of the patient's physical limitations and associated anorexia, laxatives are generally the mainstay of treatment.

Knowledge of the different classes of laxatives (Box 4.B) and the composition of various preparations (Box 4.C) permits rational combinations to be used (Figure 4.1). The best starting point varies from patient to patient. Sometimes it is appropriate to rely entirely on rectal measures or just to use a faecal softener, as in most patients with inoperable bowel obstruction.

Box 4.B   Classification of laxatives

Bulk-forming drugs (fibre)
Ispaghula husk (e.g. Fybogel,
    Regulan)
Methylcellulose
Sterculia (e.g. Normacol)

Osmotic laxatives
Lactulose syrup
Liquid paraffin and magnesium hydroxide
    emulsion BP
Macrogols (polyethylene glycols)
Magnesium hydroxide suspension
    (Milk of Magnesia)
Magnesium sulphate (Epsom Salts)

Lubricants
Liquid paraffin/mineral oil

Surface wetting agents
Docusate sodium
Poloxamer

Contact (stimulant) laxatives
Bisacodyl
Dantron
Senna
Sodium picosulphate

Box 4.C   Composition of laxatives (UK)

Bulk-forming drugs
Fybogel (sachet) ⎫
Regulan (sachet) ⎭   Ispaghula husk 3.4–6.4g
Normacol granules   Sterculia 6.2g/10g
Normacol plus granules   Sterculia 6.2g/10g + frangula 800mg/10g
Celevac tablet   Methylcellulose 500mg

continued

Box 4.C   Continued

Surface wetting agents
Docusate sodium syrup 50mg/5ml[a]
Docusate sodium tablet 100mg[a]

Osmotic agents
Lactulose syrup 3.35g/5ml
Movicol sachet   Macrogols (polyethylene glycols) 3350
Liquid paraffin and magnesium   Magnesium hydroxide mixture BP
   hydroxide emulsion BP (10ml)   7.5ml + liquid paraffin 2.5ml
Milk of Magnesia suspension (5ml)   Magnesium hydroxide 350mg
Epsom Salts crystals (5ml)
        solution (10ml)   Magnesium sulphate 4g

Contact (stimulant) laxatives
Standardised senna tablet 7.5mg
Bisacodyl tablet 5mg
Bisacodyl suppository 5mg, 10mg
Sodium picosulphate syrup 5mg/5ml
Co-danthrusate suspension   Dantron 50mg + docusate sodium 60mg
   (5ml)/capsule
Co-danthramer suspension   Dantron 25mg + poloxamer 200mg
   (5ml)/capsule
Co-danthramer strong capsule   Dantron 37.5mg + poloxamer 500mg
Co-danthramer strong suspension   Dantron 75mg + poloxamer 1g
   (5ml)

---

a. docusate enhances the absorption of liquid paraffin; combined preparations of
these substances are prohibited in some countries.

Opioid-induced constipation

Opioids cause constipation by decreasing propulsive intestinal activity and
increasing non-propulsive activity, and also by enhancing the absorption
of fluid and electrolytes. Colonic contact laxatives reduce intestinal ring
contractions and thereby facilitate propulsive activity; they provide a logical
approach to the correction of opioid-induced constipation.

Patients receiving an opioid often need a higher dose of a contact (stimulant)
laxative than that recommended for general use by the manufacturers. In
the UK, most palliative care units use co-danthrusate or co-danthramer, i.e. a
combination of a stimulant laxative (dantron) and a faecal softener (Box 4.D).
Alternatively senna 15mg or bisacodyl 10mg and docusate tablets 100–200mg
can be used concurrently o.n.–t.d.s.

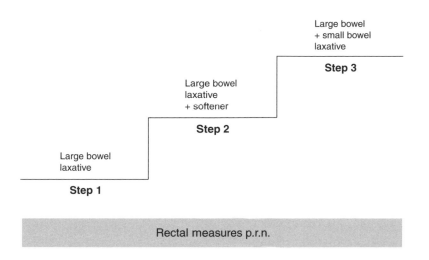

Figure 4.1   A therapeutic step-ladder with safety net (rectal measures) for drug-induced constipation. Doses should be titrated upwards as necessary, e.g. bisacodyl 10mg o.n.–t.d.s. PO on step 1. Many centres begin on step 2 (see p.112).

Note:

- bulk-forming drugs have little to offer in the management of opioid-induced constipation, and sometimes make matters worse
- many patients prescribed lactulose for opioid-induced constipation remain constipated; examination may demonstrate palpable 'faecal porridge' in the caecum and 'faecal rock cakes' in the descending colon, thereby emphasising the need to enhance colonic propulsion
- about 1/3 of patients receiving morphine will need rectal measures (laxative suppositories, enemas, digital evacuation) either regularly or intermittently.

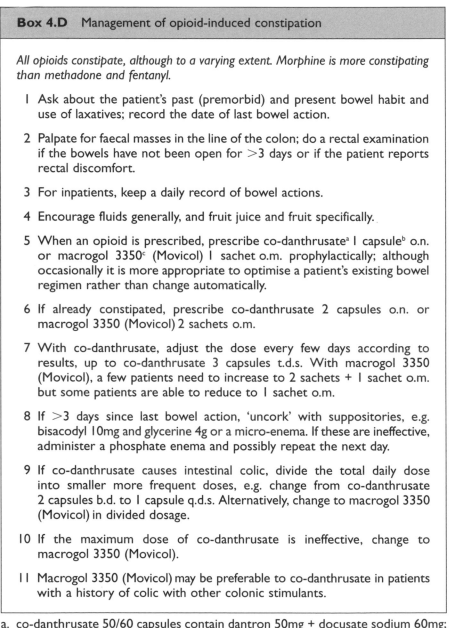

Box 4.D   Management of opioid-induced constipation

All opioids constipate, although to a varying extent. Morphine is more constipating than methadone and fentanyl.

1   Ask about the patient's past (premorbid) and present bowel habit and use of laxatives; record the date of last bowel action.

2   Palpate for faecal masses in the line of the colon; do a rectal examination if the bowels have not been open for >3 days or if the patient reports rectal discomfort.

3   For inpatients, keep a daily record of bowel actions.

4   Encourage fluids generally, and fruit juice and fruit specifically.

5   When an opioid is prescribed, prescribe co-danthrusate[a] 1 capsule[b] o.n. or macrogol 3350[c] (Movicol) 1 sachet o.m. prophylactically; although occasionally it is more appropriate to optimise a patient's existing bowel regimen rather than change automatically.

6   If already constipated, prescribe co-danthrusate 2 capsules o.n. or macrogol 3350 (Movicol) 2 sachets o.m.

7   With co-danthrusate, adjust the dose every few days according to results, up to co-danthrusate 3 capsules t.d.s. With macrogol 3350 (Movicol), a few patients need to increase to 2 sachets + 1 sachet o.m. but some patients are able to reduce to 1 sachet o.m.

8   If >3 days since last bowel action, 'uncork' with suppositories, e.g. bisacodyl 10mg and glycerine 4g or a micro-enema. If these are ineffective, administer a phosphate enema and possibly repeat the next day.

9   If co-danthrusate causes intestinal colic, divide the total daily dose into smaller more frequent doses, e.g. change from co-danthrusate 2 capsules b.d. to 1 capsule q.d.s. Alternatively, change to macrogol 3350 (Movicol) in divided dosage.

10   If the maximum dose of co-danthrusate is ineffective, change to macrogol 3350 (Movicol).

11   Macrogol 3350 (Movicol) may be preferable to co-danthrusate in patients with a history of colic with other colonic stimulants.

a.   co-danthrusate 50/60 capsules contain dantron 50mg + docusate sodium 60mg; dantron is a colonic stimulant and docusate is a surface wetting agent/faecal softener

b.   alternatively, supply co-danthrusate suspension (5ml = 1 capsule)

c.   macrogol 3350 (Movicol) is an osmotic laxative.

Dyspepsia

Dyspepsia ('indigestion') is discomfort or pain in the upper abdomen, particularly after meals, generally related to a functional or an organic disorder of the stomach or duodenum.

Causes

There are many causes of dyspepsia (Box 4.E). From a therapeutic perspective in advanced cancer, dyspepsia can be divided into four categories:

- small stomach capacity
- gassy
- acid
- dysmotility.

Box 4.E Causes of dyspepsia in advanced cancer

Cancer
Small stomach capacity
   large unresected stomach cancer
   massive ascites
Gastroparesis (paraneoplastic
   visceral neuropathy)

Treatment
Postsurgical
   postgastrectomy
   reflux oesophagitis
Radiotherapy
   lumbar spine
   epigastrium
Drugs
   physical irritant → gastritis, e.g.
     iron, tranexamic acid
   acid stimulant → gastritis, e.g.
     NSAIDs, corticosteroids
   delayed gastric emptying, e.g.
     antimuscarinics, opioids, cisplatin

Debility
Oesophageal candidiasis
Minimal food and fluid intake
Anxiety → aerophagia

Concurrent
Organic dyspepsia
   peptic ulcer
   reflux oesophagitis
   cholelithiasis
   renal failure
Non-ulcer dyspepsia
   dysmotility
   aerophagia

Functional dyspepsia (dyspepsia without apparent organic cause) is generally caused by dysmotility. It is seen in about 25% of the general population and is therefore common in patients with cancer.

Many cases of 'squashed stomach syndrome'[17] and 'cancer-associated dyspepsia syndrome'[18] are probably cases of functional dyspepsia and/or gastric stasis (*see* below) exacerbated by:

- hepatomegaly
- gross ascites.

Evaluation

It is important to differentiate between the four types of dyspepsia because the treatment differs. Careful history taking generally indicates which type is predominant. Patients with dysmotility may also have symptoms or a history of irritable bowel syndrome.

Management

Small stomach capacity

If dyspepsia is associated with a small stomach capacity, patients should be advised to separate their main fluid from their solid intake, and to eat 'small and often', i.e. take 5–6 small meals/snacks during the day rather than 2–3 big meals.

Patients with a small stomach capacity may benefit from an antiflatulent after meals, to help clear space in an overfull stomach.

Gassy dyspepsia

Prescribe an antiflatulent, e.g. dimeticone. This is available on its own but may conveniently be given in the form of Asilone, a proprietary antacid. Depending on a patient's individual needs, this can be given p.r.n., q.d.s. or both.

Acid dyspepsia

Prescribe an antacid, an H_2-receptor antagonist (e.g. cimetidine, ranitidine) or a proton pump inhibitor (e.g. lansoprazole, omeprazole). A proton pump inhibitor should also be used in cases of NSAID-related gastritis.[19,20]

Dysmotility dyspepsia

This is not helped by gastric acid reduction. Prescribe metoclopramide to normalise disordered gastric motility.

Gastric stasis

Gastric stasis resulting in delayed gastric emptying is common in advanced cancer. It is probably the main causal factor in about 25% of cases of nausea and vomiting.[21]

Clinical features

The clinical features of gastric stasis range from mild dyspepsia and anorexia to persistent severe nausea and large-volume vomiting (Box 4.F). Gastric stasis is normally functional and is associated with one or more of the following conditions:

- dysmotility dyspepsia (often longstanding)
- constipation[22]
- drugs (e.g. opioids, antimuscarinics, aluminium hydroxide, levodopa)
- cancer of the head of the pancreas (disrupts duodenal transit)
- paraneoplastic autonomic neuropathy
- retroperitoneal disease (→ nerve dysfunction)
- spinal cord compression
- diabetic autonomic neuropathy.

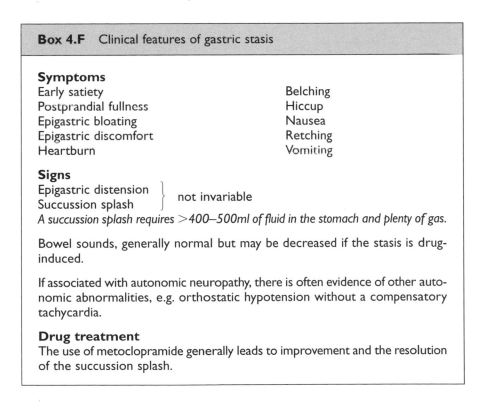

Box 4.F   Clinical features of gastric stasis

Symptoms

Early satiety	Belching
Postprandial fullness	Hiccup
Epigastric bloating	Nausea
Epigastric discomfort	Retching
Heartburn	Vomiting

Signs

Epigastric distension ⎫ not invariable
Succussion splash ⎭
A succussion splash requires >400–500ml of fluid in the stomach and plenty of gas.

Bowel sounds, generally normal but may be decreased if the stasis is drug-induced.

If associated with autonomic neuropathy, there is often evidence of other autonomic abnormalities, e.g. orthostatic hypotension without a compensatory tachycardia.

Drug treatment
The use of metoclopramide generally leads to improvement and the resolution of the succussion splash.

Management

Management comprises explanation and the use of a prokinetic drug, e.g. metoclopramide (Figure 4.2). As a general rule, *prokinetic and antimuscarinic drugs should not be prescribed concurrently.* Antimuscarinics block cholinergic receptors on intestinal muscle fibres,[23] and thereby competitively block the effect of prokinetics. However, domperidone and metoclopramide will still exert an antagonistic effect at the dopamine type 2 receptors in the chemoreceptor trigger zone (area postrema) in the brain stem.

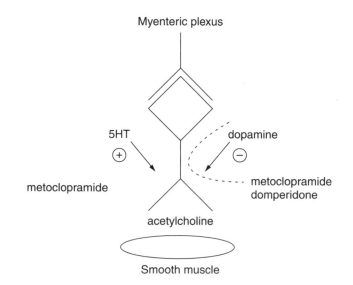

Figure 4.2   Schematic representation of drug effects on antroduodenal co-ordination via a postganglionic effect on the cholinergic nerves from the myenteric plexus.
⊕ stimulatory effect of 5HT triggered by metoclopramide; ⊖ inhibitory effect of dopamine; ----- blockade of dopamine inhibition by metoclopramide and domperidone.

Metoclopramide, with its dual mode of action, is generally preferable; it is available both in oral formulations and injections. However, because it does not cross the blood-brain barrier, domperidone should be used in patients with parkinsonism in whom central dopamine type 2 receptor antagonism is likely to be detrimental.

Gastric outflow obstruction

Delayed gastric emptying is sometimes associated with an organic obstruction:

● cancer of the gastric antrum
● external compression of the gastric antrum or duodenum by a tumour.

If severe, this causes major difficulties in management. Each case needs individual evaluation and treatment. In most cases, the obstruction is not complete. Even with no oral intake, the stomach needs to clear:

- swallowed saliva (normally 1500ml/24h)
- basal gastric juices (1500ml/24h).

Thus, if a patient is vomiting less than 2–3L/24h, something is getting past the obstruction.

An antimuscarinic with both antisecretory and antispasmodic properties should be prescribed, e.g. hyoscine *butylbromide* 80–120mg/24h by CSCI. This approximately halves gastric secretions and will also reduce salivary volume.[24] In countries where parenteral hyoscine *butylbromide* is not available, glycopyrronium 600–1200microgram/24h can be substituted.

Somatostatin analogues which are antisecretory but not antispasmodic are used at some centres e.g. octreotide 300–600microgram/24h.[25] Their cost is a potentially limiting factor. A venting procedure is occasionally necessary, e.g. nasogastric tube or gastrostomy.

Nausea and vomiting

Nausea and vomiting occurs in about 50% of patients with advanced cancer. Gastric stasis (*see* p.114), bowel obstruction (*see* p.120), drugs and bio chemical abnormalities account for most cases. The sequence of events, together with an appropriate level of suspicion, often suggests the probable cause.

It is important to identify the most likely cause(s) in each patient because the treatment is dependent on the cause. On the basis of putative sites of action, it is possible to derive anti-emetic drugs of choice for different situations (Box 4.G).

Corticosteroids possibly act by reducing the permeability of the chemoreceptor trigger zone and of the blood-brain barrier to emetogenic substances, and by reducing the neuronal content of gamma-aminobutyric acid (GABA) in the brain stem.[26] In obstruction, a corticosteroid may also help by reducing inflammation at the site of the block, and thereby increase the lumen. Further, by reducing pressure on intestinal nerves, the use of a corticosteroid may correct neural dysfunction and the associated functional obstruction.

Box 4.G   Management of nausea and vomiting in palliative care

1 After clinical evaluation, document the most likely cause(s) of the nausea and vomiting in the patient's case notes, e.g. gastric stasis, intestinal obstruction, biochemical, drugs, raised intracranial pressure.
2 Ask the patient to record symptoms and response to treatment, preferably using a diary.
3 Correct correctable causes/exacerbating factors, e.g. drugs, severe pain, infection, cough, hypercalcaemia. *(Correction of hypercalcaemia is not always appropriate in a dying patient.)* Anxiety exacerbates nausea and vomiting from any cause and may need specific treatment.
4 Prescribe the most appropriate anti-emetic stat, regularly and p.r.n. *(see below).* Give by SC injection if continuous nausea or frequent vomiting, preferably by CSCI.

Commonly used anti-emetics

Prokinetic anti-emetic (about 50% of prescriptions)
For gastritis, gastric stasis, functional bowel obstruction (peristaltic failure):
metoclopramide 10mg PO (orally) stat & q.d.s. or 10mg SC stat & 40–100mg/24h CSCI, & 10mg p.r.n. up to q.d.s.

Anti-emetic acting principally in chemoreceptor trigger zone (about 25% of prescriptions)
For most chemical causes of vomiting, e.g. morphine, hypercalcaemia, renal failure:
haloperidol 1.5–3mg PO stat & o.n. or 2.5–5mg SC stat & 2.5–10mg/24h CSCI, & 2.5–5mg p.r.n. up to q.d.s.
Metoclopramide also has a central action.

Antispasmodic and antisecretory anti-emetic
If bowel colic and/or need to reduce gastro-intestinal secretions:
hyoscine *butylbromide* 20mg SC stat, 80–200mg/24h CSCI, & 20mg SC hourly p.r.n.

Anti-emetic acting principally in the vomiting centre
For raised intracranial pressure (in conjunction with dexamethasone), motion sickness and in organic bowel obstruction:
cyclizine 50mg PO stat & b.d.–t.d.s. or 50mg SC stat & 100–150mg/24h CSCI, & 50mg p.r.n. up to q.d.s.

Broad-spectrum anti-emetic
For organic bowel obstruction and when other anti-emetics are unsatisfactory:
levomepromazine (methotrimeprazine) 6–12.5mg PO/SC stat, o.n. & p.r.n. up to q.d.s.

5 Review anti-emetic dose every 24h, taking note of p.r.n. use and the patient's diary.
6 If little benefit despite optimising the dose, have you got the cause right?
   • if no, change to an alternative anti-emetic and optimise
   • if yes, provided the anti-emetic has been optimised, add or substitute a second anti-emetic.

continued

7 Anti-emetics for inoperable bowel obstruction are best given by CSCI. Levomepromazine (methotrimeprazine) is the exception; it can be given as a single SC dose o.n.:

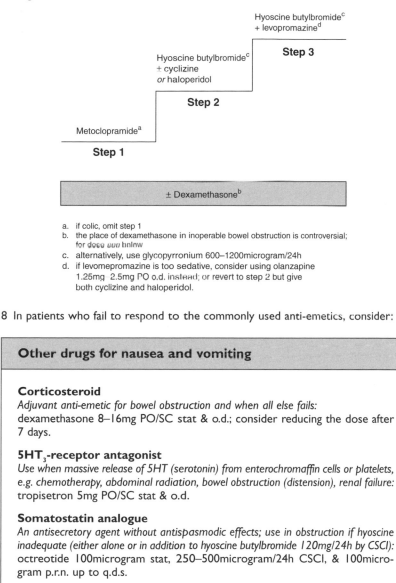

Hyoscine butylbromide[c]
+ levopromazine[d]

Step 3

Hyoscine butylbromide[c]
+ cyclizine
or haloperidol

Step 2

Metoclopramide[a]

Step 1

± Dexamethasone[b]

a. if colic, omit step 1
b. the place of dexamethasone in inoperable bowel obstruction is controversial; for dose see below
c. alternatively, use glycopyrronium 600–1200microgram/24h
d. if levomepromazine is too sedative, consider using olanzapine 1.25mg–2.5mg PO o.d. instead; or revert to step 2 but give both cyclizine and haloperidol.

8 In patients who fail to respond to the commonly used anti-emetics, consider:

Other drugs for nausea and vomiting

Corticosteroid
Adjuvant anti-emetic for bowel obstruction and when all else fails:
dexamethasone 8–16mg PO/SC stat & o.d.; consider reducing the dose after 7 days.

5HT$_3$-receptor antagonist
Use when massive release of 5HT (serotonin) from enterochromaffin cells or platelets, e.g. chemotherapy, abdominal radiation, bowel obstruction (distension), renal failure:
tropisetron 5mg PO/SC stat & o.d.

Somatostatin analogue
An antisecretory agent without antispasmodic effects; use in obstruction if hyoscine inadequate (either alone or in addition to hyoscine butylbromide 120mg/24h by CSCI):
octreotide 100microgram stat, 250–500microgram/24h CSCI, & 100microgram p.r.n. up to q.d.s.

 9 Some patients with nausea and vomiting need more than one anti-emetic.
10 *Antimuscarinic drugs block the cholinergic pathway through which prokinetics act; concurrent use antagonises the prokinetic effect of metoclopramide and is best avoided.*
11 Continue anti-emetics unless the cause is self-limiting.
12 Except in organic bowel obstruction, consider changing to PO after 72h of good control with CSCI.

Obstruction

The focus here is on patients for whom available anticancer treatments have been exhausted. Obstruction of the alimentary tract can occur at any level. At each level, the obstruction can be functional (paralytic) or organic (mechanical), or both. It can also be partial or complete, and transient (acute) or persistent (chronic).

Organic oesophageal obstruction, manifests as dysphagia for solids first and liquids second. It is normally managed by palliative surgery (e.g. LASER therapy), insertion of an endo-oesophageal tube or palliative radiotherapy.

Gastric outlet and small bowel obstruction are associated with frequent, large volume vomits; whereas with large bowel obstruction (and possibly distal small bowel), vomiting may well be limited to later in the day. However, in advanced cancer, there are commonly multiple sites of obstruction involving both small and large bowel. In most cases the obstruction is *not* complete.

Causes

Bowel obstruction in advanced cancer may be caused by one or more of the following:

- the cancer itself
- past treatment, e.g. adhesions, postradiation ischaemic fibrosis
- drugs, e.g. opioids, antimuscarinics
- associated with debility, e.g. constipation
- an unrelated benign condition, e.g. strangulated hernia.

Clinical features of chronic bowel obstruction

In *acute* bowel obstruction there is typically a single discrete lesion, whereas in *chronic* obstruction (persistent or remittent) there may well be several sites of partial obstruction in both small and large bowels. Retroperitoneal disease may cause visceral neuropathy and functional obstruction. In consequence, the quartet of symptoms and signs which point to a diagnosis of *acute* intestinal obstruction (abdominal distension, pain, vomiting and constipation) is often not so obvious in *chronic* obstruction in advanced cancer. For example, distension may be minimal because of multiple intra-abdominal malignant adhesions. Bowel sounds vary from absent to overactive with borborygmi; *tinkling bowel sounds are unusual*. Some patients have diarrhoea rather than constipation.

Surgical management

The following are all contra-indications to surgical intervention:

- previous laparotomy findings preclude the prospect of a successful intervention
- intra-abdominal carcinomatosis as evidenced by diffuse palpable intra-abdominal tumours
- massive ascites which re-accumulates rapidly after paracentesis.[27]

In addition, weight loss of >9kg is associated with a poor outcome after surgery.[28]

Surgical intervention should be considered if the following criteria are *all* fulfilled:

- a single discrete organic obstruction seems likely, e.g. postoperative adhesions or an isolated neoplasm
- the patient's general condition is good, i.e. he does not have widely disseminated disease, has been independent and active, and weight loss is <9kg
- the patient is willing to undergo surgery.

Medical management

In patients in whom an operative approach is contra-indicated, it is generally possible to relieve symptoms adequately with drugs.[28] A nasogastric tube and IV hydration are rarely necessary.

Management focuses primarily on the relief of nausea and vomiting. For those without colic and who are still passing flatus, a prokinetic is the initial drug of choice. For patients with severe colic, prokinetics are contra-indicated. Instead prescribe an antisecretory and antispasmodic drug, e.g. hyoscine *butylbromide* or glycopyrronium (Box 4.G).

Bulk-forming, osmotic and stimulant laxatives should also be stopped. A series of drug changes over several days may be necessary before optimum relief is achieved. For the constant background cancer pain, morphine or diamorphine should be given regularly. If the patient is receiving parenteral metoclopramide or hyoscine *butylbromide*, the opioid can also be given by CSCI.

A phosphate enema should be given if constipation is a probable contributory factor and a faecal softener prescribed, i.e. docusate sodium tablets 100–200mg b.d.

Corticosteroids benefit some patients with inoperable bowel obstruction.[29] Because spontaneous resolution occurs in at least 1/3 of patients, it is important not to prescribe a corticosteroid too soon. Treat the symptoms as suggested above and then, after 7–10 days, if the obstruction has not settled, a trial of a corticosteroid for 3 days should be considered, e.g. dexamethasone 10mg SC.[30] If there is improvement, either continue with the corticosteroid at a lower dose PO or stop and review the need for long-term treatment.

Consider adding octreotide if hyoscine *butylbromide* 120–200mg by CSCI fails to relieve the vomiting.[25] Octreotide has an antisecretory effect throughout the alimentary tract. Octreotide can also be given by CSCI, e.g. 250–500microgram/24h, occasionally more. A reduction in intestinal contents reduces distension and thereby the likelihood of colic and vomiting.

Because raised intraluminal pressure results in the release of 5HT (serotonin) from the enterochromaffin cells in the bowel wall, some patients benefit from a $5HT_3$-receptor antagonist, e.g. granisetron, ondansetron, tropisetron.

A venting gastrostomy is rarely necessary for chronic obstruction in advanced cancer.[31] Indeed, patients managed by drug therapy should be encouraged to drink and eat small amounts of their favourite beverages and food. Some patients find that they can manage food best in the morning.

Antimuscarinics and diminished fluid intake result in a dry mouth and thirst. These are generally relieved by conscientious mouth care. A few ml of fluid every 30min, possibly administered as a small ice cube, often brings relief. IV hydration is rarely needed.

Respiratory symptoms

Breathlessness

Breathlessness is the subjective experience of breathing discomfort. It is present in 70% of patients with cancer in the last few weeks before death, and is severe in 25% of patients in the last week of life.[32] Breathlessness:

- is often intermittent, occurring in episodes lasting 5–15min precipitated by exertion, bending over, or even just talking, and is associated with feelings of exhaustion
- restricts activities, leading to a loss of independence and of role, and resulting in frustration, anger and depression[33]
- induces feelings of anxiety (particularly when present at rest), fear, panic and impending death (Figure 4.3).[34]

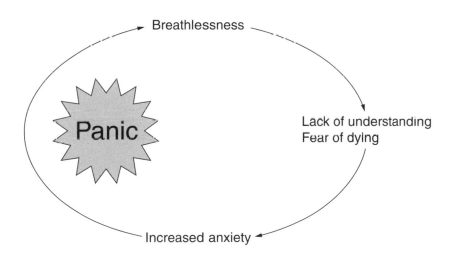

Figure 4.3   Breathlessness is a common trigger for panic.[34]

Breathlessness is generally associated with an increased respiratory rate. If the resting respiratory rate is 30–35/min, activity or anxiety may increase this to 50–60/min.

Causes

Breathlessness in advanced cancer is generally multifactorial (Box 4.H). Many patients have weak inspiratory muscles. About half are hypoxic, and about 20% have evidence of concurrent cardiac disease.[35]

Box 4.H   Causes of breathlessness in advanced cancer

Cancer
Pleural effusion(s)
Obstruction of a large airway
Replacement of lung by cancer
Lymphangitis carcinomatosa
Tumour cell micro-emboli
Pericardial effusion
Phrenic nerve palsy
SVC obstruction
Massive ascites
Abdominal distension
Cachexia-anorexia syndrome
    respiratory muscle weakness

Treatment
Pneumonectomy
Radiation-induced fibrosis
Chemotherapy-induced
    pneumonitis
    fibrosis
    cardiomyopathy
Progestogens
    stimulate ventilation
    increase sensitivity to carbon dioxide

Debility
Anaemia
Atelectasis
Pulmonary embolism
Pneumonia
Empyema
Muscle weakness

Concurrent
COPD
Asthma
Heart failure
Acidosis
Fever
Pneumothorax
Panic disorder, anxiety,
    depression

Management

Unless investigation reveals remediable causes, breathlessness in advanced cancer can be divided into three categories:

- breathlessness on exertion (prognosis = months-to-years)
- breathlessness at rest (prognosis = weeks-to-months)
- terminal breathlessness (prognosis = days-to-weeks).

The relative importance of the three treatment categories (*correct the correctable, non-drug treatment, drug treatment*) changes as the patient's condition deteriorates (Figure 4.4).

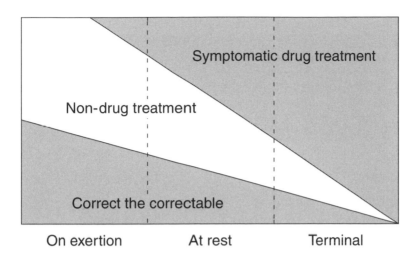

Figure 4.4   Treatment for severe breathlessness at different stages in advanced cancer.

Correct the correctable
Particularly while the patient is still ambulant, consideration should be given to the identification and correction of correctable causes (Table 4.2).

Bronchospasm is not always associated with wheeze, particularly in patients with a history of chronic asthma, chronic bronchitis or heavy smoking. A peak flow meter should be used to diagnose bronchospasm, testing before and after a standard dose of an inhaled nebulised β-adrenoceptor agonist (sympathomimetic), e.g. salbutamol.

Non-drug treatment
Non-drug treatment begins by exploring the patient's experience of breath-lessness (Box 4.1). Open acknowledgement of the fear and feelings of terror and panic associated with the acute exacerbations, e.g. when climbing stairs, is the key to enable the patient (and the family) to cope. The patient must be assured that they will not die during an attack; emphasise that 'Although you may feel you're suffocating, you've always recovered, and you always will'.

Generally, the breathless patient should be referred to a physiotherapist for breathing retraining and advice about activity pacing; this is particularly important when the patient is experiencing panic attacks.[36]

Symptomatic drug treatment
Symptomatic drug treatment for breathlessness should be used only after non-drug treatments have been fully exploited (Figure 4.5).

Table 4.2   Correctable causes of breathlessness

Cause	Treatment
Respiratory infection	Antibiotics
	Physiotherapy
COPD/asthma	Bronchodilators
	Corticosteroids
	Physiotherapy
Hypoxia	Trial of oxygen
Obstruction of bronchus, or superior vena cava	Corticosteroids
	Radiotherapy
	Stent
	LASER (bronchus only)
Lymphangitis carcinomatosa	Corticosteroids
	Diuretics
	Bronchodilators
Pleural effusion	Thoracocentesis
	Drainage and pleurodesis
Ascites	Diuretics (see p.141)
	Paracentesis
Pericardial effusion	Paracentesis
	Corticosteroids
Anaemia	Blood transfusion
	Epoetin
Cardiac failure	Diuretics
	ACE inhibitors
Pulmonary embolism	Anticoagulation

Salbutamol (and theophylline) increase muscle strength, and therefore may be beneficial in the absence of reversible bronchospasm.[37]

Morphine reduces the respiratory drive:

- if on morphine for pain, increase the dose by 30–50%
- if not on oral morphine, 5–6mg q4h–q6h is a good starting dose.

Do not give morphine by nebuliser; *nebulised morphine is no better than nebulised saline.*[38]

Box 4.1 Non-drug treatment of breathlessness

Overt discussion of the patient's and the family's concerns
Explain the cause(s) of the breathlessness, and explore anxiety about it.
Assure that breathlessness in itself is not damaging or life-threatening.
Emphasise that the patient will not die during an acute exacerbation.
Help the patient to adjust to the loss of physical abilities and roles.

General measures

Activity pacing, i.e. eat, rest, wash, rest, dress, rest, etc.
Help with housework
Sit to do tasks, e.g. washing, shaving
Bed downstairs
Space around bed

Loose clothing around neck
Avoid very hot environment
Open window/cool draught
Use of electric fan
Cold wet flannel wiped over face

Physiotherapy
Breathing advice and exercises, e.g. breathing out slowly through pursed lips
can help patients with expiratory obstruction.
Encourage exertion to breathlessness to increase tolerance to breathlessness and maintain fitness.
Relaxation therapy/techniques:
● slow regular deep breathing
● relax shoulders, back, neck and arms/massage
● visualisation.

Additional measures
Acupuncture
Art/music therapy

Attend day centre
Respite admissions

Diazepam can be given if the patient remains very anxious despite non-drug
measures, and use of oral morphine:

● 5–10mg stat and o.n.; in the very elderly, 2–5mg
● reduce the dose after several days if the patient becomes drowsy.

Patients who continue to experience panic may also need diazepam 2–5mg
p.r.n. Some centres use lorazepam 1mg *sublingually* b.d. and p.r.n. In relatively
long-term situations, an SSRI may be helpful, either alone or in combination.[39]

Oxygen
Oxygen therapy increases alveolar oxygen tension and decreases the work
of breathing necessary to maintain a given arterial oxygen tension. The concentration given varies with the underlying condition:

● 60% in asthma, pneumonia, pulmonary embolism, fibrosing alveolitis
● 28% in hypercapnic ventilatory failure, e.g. COPD.

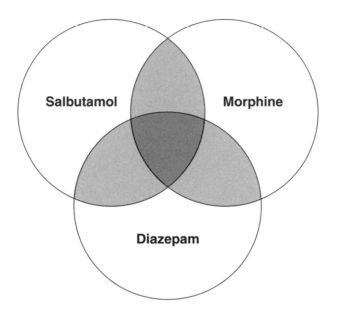

Figure 4.5   Drugs for the symptomatic relief of breathlessness.

Patients with hypercapnic ventilatory failure who are dependent upon hypoxia for their respiratory drive should not be given a high concentration. Inappropriate prescription can have serious or fatal effects.

Oxygen is often beneficial in patients with breathlessness at rest, particularly if hypoxic. It is best given by nasal prongs (4L/min) because these do not interfere with social contact. Oxygen does not always help and should be continued only if there is clear benefit. Patients should be asked to compare nasal oxygen with both an electric fan and a draught through an open window.

A low initial oxygen saturation does not necessarily mean oxygen will help. A pulse oximeter can be used to identify patients whose oxygen saturation is objectively improved by oxygen. In patients with severe breathlessness on exertion, there may be a place for a trial of oxygen before activity, e.g. 4L/min for 5min.

Terminal breathlessness

Patients often fear suffocating to death. A positive approach to the patient and their family about the relief of terminal breathlessness is therefore important:

- no patient should die with distressing breathlessness

- failure to relieve terminal breathlessness is a failure to utilise drug treatment correctly
- give an opioid with a sedative-anxiolytic by CSCI, and SC p.r.n., e.g. diamorphine/morphine with midazolam
- if the patient becomes agitated or confused (sometimes aggravated by midazolam), haloperidol should be added (see p.171).

Patients and their carers generally accept that drowsiness may need to be the price paid for greater comfort.

Unless there is overwhelming persistent distress despite the above measures, deep sedation to keep the patient unaware around the clock is *not* the aim of treatment (see p.158). Indeed, some patients become mentally brighter when the breathlessness is reduced. However, because increasing drowsiness is generally a feature of the deteriorating clinical condition, it is important to explain the aim of treatment to the family (i.e. relief of distress) and also to stress the gravity of the situation.

Death rattle

Death rattle is a term used to describe a rattling noise produced by secretions in the hypopharynx oscillating in time with inspiration and expiration. Generally death rattle is seen only in patients who are extremely weak and close to death. It occurs in 30–50% of patients and is distressing for relatives, carers and other patients.[40]

Management

Non-drug treatment
The most effective measure for easing the family's disquiet is explanation that the semi-conscious or unconscious patient is not distressed by the rattle.[40] Position the patient in a semi-prone position to encourage postural drainage. Most patients are distressed by suctioning; generally this should be reserved for unconscious patients.

Drug treatment
An antimuscarinic antisecretory drug needs to be given promptly because it does not affect existing pharyngeal secretions (Table 4.3).[41] The rattle is reduced in 1/2–2/3 of patients.[40]

Antimuscarinics are probably most effective for rattle associated with the pooling of saliva in the pharynx ('real death rattle') and least effective for rattle caused by bronchial secretions (as a result of infection or oedema) or related

Table 4.3 Antisecretory drugs for death rattle

Drug	Stat SC dose	CSCI/24h
Hyoscine *hydrobromide*	0.4–0.6mg	1.2–2.4mg
Hyoscine *butylbromide*	20mg	20–40mg
Glycopyrronium	0.2–0.4mg	0.6–1.2mg

to the reflux of gastric contents ('pseudo death rattle').[42] Hyoscine *hydrobromide* crosses the blood-brain barrier and possesses additional anti-emetic and sedative properties.

Acute tracheal compression/massive haemorrhage into trachea

This is a rare palliative care emergency:

- IV diazepam/midazolam 5–20mg until the patient is unconscious
- PR diazepam or IM midazolam 20mg, if IV administration not possible
- continuous company.

Cough

Causes include:

- smoking
- asthma
- COPD
- chest infection
- acid reflux
- heart failure
- intrathoracic cancer
- ACE inhibitor (<10%).

Management

Correct the correctable
Specific treatment for underlying cause, e.g.:

- bronchodilators
- antibiotics.

Non-drug treatment

- advise how to cough effectively; it is hard to cough effectively lying on your back
- physiotherapy, including postural drainage
- steam or chemical inhalations.

Drug treatment
Symptomatic drug treatment (Box 4.J) depends on the aim of treatment:

- aid expectoration if a wet (productive) cough and the patient is able to cough effectively (Figure 4.6)
- suppress expectoration if a dry (non-productive) cough or the patient is too weak to cough effectively (Figure 4.7).

Box 4.J Drugs for cough

Protussives
Topical mucolytics
Nebulised 0.9% saline
Chemical inhalations
   compound benzoin tincture
    (Friar's balsam)
   carbol
   menthol and eucalyptus

Irritant mucolytics, e.g.
Guaifenesin
Ipecacuanha
Potassium iodide

Chemical mucolytics
Acetylcysteine (not UK)
Carbocisteine

Antitussives
Peripheral
Simple linctus (a 'demulcent')
Benzonatate (not UK)
Nebulised bupivacaine
  (rarely used)

Central
Opioid derivatives
  dextromethorphan
  levopropoxyphene (not UK)
  pholcodine

Opioids
  codeine
  hydrocodone (not UK)
  hydromorphone
  morphine

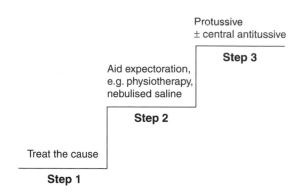

Figure 4.6 Treatment ladder for wet (productive) cough. Step 3: the antitussive reduces the frequency of coughing, while the protussive makes the coughing more effective.

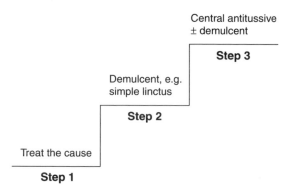

Figure 4.7 Treatment ladder for dry (non-productive) cough and for a patient who is too weak to cough effectively.

Hiccup

Hiccup is a pathological reflex characterised by spasm of the diaphragm, resulting in sudden inspiration followed by abrupt closure of the glottis.

Causes

In advanced cancer, causes include:

- gastric distension (common)
- gastro-oesophageal reflux
- diaphragmatic irritation
- infection
- uraemia
- phrenic nerve irritation (rare)
- CNS tumour (rare).

Acute management options

Pharyngeal stimulation
Oropharyngeal stimulation activates a neural 'gating' mechanism. Although not commonly used by clinicians, awareness of these options is sometimes useful:

- drinking from 'wrong' side of a cup or cold key down back of neck (acts via hyperextension of neck)
- granulated sugar (2 heaped teaspoons) or liqueur (2 glasses) rapidly ingested
- pulling the tongue forcibly out of the mouth
- massage of the junction between hard and soft palate with a cotton bob
- nebulised saline (2ml of 0.9% saline over 5min).[43]

Reduce gastric distension
Gastric distension probably accounts for most cases. Consider:

- peppermint water, this facilitates belching by relaxing the lower oesophageal sphincter (an old-fashioned remedy)
- dimeticone, an antiflatulent contained in some proprietary antacids, e.g. Asilone or Maalox Plus 10ml
- metoclopramide 10mg, tightens the lower oesophageal sphincter and hastens gastric emptying.

Elevation of pCO_2
This inhibits processing of the hiccup reflex in the brain stem:

- rebreathing from a paper bag
- breath-holding.

Muscle relaxant (and central suppressant effect)

- baclofen 5mg PO
- nifedipine 10mg PO/SL
- midazolam 2mg IV, followed by 1–2mg increments every 3–5min.

Central suppression of hiccup reflex

- haloperidol 5–10mg PO or IV if no response
- chlorpromazine 10–25mg PO or IV if no response
- sodium valproate 200–500mg PO or IV if no response.

Maintenance treatment

Gastric distension

- dimeticone, e.g. Asilone or Maalox Plus 10ml q.d.s.
- metoclopramide 10mg q.d.s.

Gastro-oesophageal reflux

- prokinetic *and/or*
- H$_2$-receptor antagonist, PPI.

Diaphragmatic irritation or other cause

- baclofen 5–20mg t.d.s., occasionally more[44]
- nifedipine 10–20mg t.d.s., occasionally more[45]
- haloperidol 1.5–3mg o.n.[46]
- sodium valproate 200–1000mg o.n.[47]
- midazolam 10–60mg/24h by CSCI if all else fails.[48]

Urinary symptoms

Useful definitions

Frequency	Passage of urine seven or more times during the day and twice or more times at night.
Urgency	A strong and sudden desire to void.
Urge incontinence	The involuntary loss of urine associated with a strong desire to void.
Detrusor instability	Detrusor contracts uninhibitedly and causes: diurnal frequency nocturnal frequency ⎤ increasing severity urgency urge incontinence ⎦ (The second most common cause of urinary incontinence in women.)

continued

Stress incontinence	The involuntary loss of urine associated with coughing, sneezing, laughing and lifting.
Genuine stress incontinence (Urethral sphincter incompetence)	The involuntary loss of urine when the intravesical pressure exceeds maximum urethral pressure in the absence of detrusor activity. The fault always lies in the sphincter mechanisms of the bladder, and is associated with multiparity, after the menopause and after hysterectomy. One or more of the following will be present: • descent of urethrovesical junction outside intra-abdominal zone of pressure • decrease in urethral pressure due to loss of urethral wall elasticity and contractility • short functional length of the urethra. (The most common cause of urinary incontinence in women.)
Dysuria	Pain during and/or after micturition. Often urethral in origin (a burning sensation) but may be caused by bladder spasm (intense suprapubic and urethral pain), or both.
Hesitancy	A prolonged delay between attempting and achieving micturition.

Urinary bladder innervation

*'You **p**ee with your **p**arasympathetics; you **s**top with your **s**ympathetics.'*

The bladder sphincter relaxes when the detrusor (bladder muscle) contracts, and vice versa (Table 4.4). The urethral sphincter is an additional voluntary mechanism innervated by the pudendal nerve (S2–4).

Table 4.4   Autonomic innervation of the bladder

Innervation	Neurotransmitter	Effect on	
		Sphincter	*Detrusor*
Sympathetic (T10–12, L1)	Noradrenaline (norepinephrine)	Contracts (α)	Relaxes (β)
Parasympathetic (S2–4)	Acetylcholine	Relaxes	Contracts

The urethra, derived embryologically from the urogenital sinus, is sensitive in women to oestrogen and progesterone. Postmenopausal urge incontinence and frequency is sometimes helped by the prescription of an oestrogen, either topically or orally. Oestrogens do not improve stress incontinence.

Effect of drugs on the bladder

Antimuscarinic drugs not only cause contraction of the bladder neck sphincter but also relax the detrusor. Detrusor sensitivity is also:

- increased by PGs
- decreased by COX inhibitors, i.e. NSAIDs.

Morphine and other opioids have several effects on bladder function:

- bladder sensation *decreased*
- sphincter tone *increased*
- detrusor tone *increased*
- ureteric tone and amplitude of contractions *increased*.

These are generally asymptomatic; occasionally hesitancy or retention occurs.

Symptoms

Common urinary symptoms in advanced cancer are:

- frequency, urgency and incontinence
- hesitancy and retention
- bladder spasms.

Causes

Causes to be considered are listed in Boxes 4.K–4.M. The causes of frequency overlap with those of urge incontinence. As in other areas of symptom management, careful evaluation is fundamental. Rectal examination to exclude faecal impaction may be necessary in debilitated/moribund patients, particularly if there is associated delirium.

Box 4.K   Causes of urgency and incontinence

Cancer
Pain
Hypercalcaemia (causes polyuria)
Intravesical ⎤ mechanical
Extravesical ⎦ irritation
Bladder spasms
Sacral plexopathy

Treatment
Radiation cystitis
Drugs
  diuretics
  cyclophosphamide
  tiaprofenic acid

Debility
Infective cystitis

Concurrent causes
Idiopathic detrusor instability
Central neurological disease
  poststroke
  multiple sclerosis
  dementia
Uraemia ⎤
Diabetes mellitus ⎬ cause polyuria
Diabetes insipidus ⎦

Box 4.L   Causes of hesitancy and retention

Cancer
Malignant enlargement of prostate
Infiltration of bladder neck
Presacral plexopathy
Spinal cord compression

Treatment
Antimuscarinics
Morphine (occasionally)
Spinal analgesia (particularly with bupivacaine)
Intrathecal nerve block

Debility
Loaded rectum
Inability to stand to void
Generalised weakness

Concurrent causes
Benign enlargement of prostate

Box 4.M   Causes of bladder spasms

Cancer
Intravesical ⎤ irritation
Extravesical ⎦

Treatment
Radiation fibrosis

Debility
Anxiety
Infective cystitis
Indwelling catheter:
    mechanical irritation by catheter balloon
    catheter sludging with partial retention

Management

Management depends on the cause, and comprises both non-drug and drug approaches. The detection and treatment of urinary infection is obviously important if it is causing dysuria, frequency and urgency.[49] 'Bladder drill' (e.g. voiding every 2h by the clock) may be helpful in someone with urge incontinence. In acute retention, check that the rectum is not impacted with faeces. If not, the following sometimes enable the person to pass urine:

- suprapubic pressure
- the sound of running water (turn a tap on)
- a hot-water bottle placed on the lower abdomen.

Drugs of choice

Urgency
Treatment may be limited by antimuscarinic effects:

- oxybutynin 2.5–5mg b.d.–q.d.s.
- tolterodine 1–2mg b.d. (more expensive, fewer adverse effects)
- amitriptyline or imipramine 25–50mg o.n.

Hesitancy

- indoramin 20mg o.n.–b.d. (initially), a selective α-1 adrenoceptor antagonist (maximum dose 100mg/24h)
- bethanechol 10–25mg b.d.–q.d.s., a muscarinic cholinergic drug.

Bladder spasms

- if catheterised, change catheter and/or reduce balloon volume
- if urinary infection
    no catheter, treat with systemic antibiotic
    catheter, treat with bladder washouts and/or urinary antiseptics, e.g. hexamine hippurate 1g b.d.
- antimuscarinic (same as for urgency)
- flavoxate 200mg t.d.s.–q.d.s. (a weak detrusor relaxant) if antimuscarinics not tolerated.

Discoloured urine

There are many causes of discoloured urine (Box 4.N). If the urine is red, it is often assumed to be haematuria, and is therefore frightening.

Box 4.N   Causes of discoloured urine

Orange/yellow
Jaundice
Nitrofurantoin

Red/pink
Beetroot
Dantron (in co-danthramer and co-danthrusate)
Doxorubicin
Haematuria
Nefopam
Phenolphthalein (in alkaline urine) present in several proprietary laxatives,
    e.g. Agarol
Rhubarb
Rifampicin

Blue
Methylene blue; present in some proprietary urinary antiseptic mixtures,
    e.g. Urised (USA)
Pseudomonas aeruginosa (pyocyanin), in alkaline urine

Dark
Metronidazole

Other symptoms

Ascites

If marked, ascites may cause a range of symptoms (Box 4.O).

Box 4.O   Clinical features of ascites

Abdominal distension	Acid reflux
Abdominal discomfort/pain	Nausea and vomiting
Inability to sit upright	Leg oedema
Early satiety	Breathlessness
Dyspepsia	Feeling of suffocation

Pathogenesis

Ascites results from an imbalance between fluid influx and efflux in the peritoneal cavity. An increased fluid influx is associated with:

● peritoneal metastases
● increased peritoneal permeability
● increased renin production secondary to raised hepatic vein pressure causing sodium and water retention which further feeds the ascitic process.

A reduced fluid efflux is associated with:

● subphrenic lymphatics blocked by tumour infiltration
● liver metastases leading to hypo-albuminaemia and possibly portal hypertension.

Management

Paracentesis
Paracentesis is appropriate for patients with a tense distended abdomen and for those who cannot tolerate spironolactone tablets (*see* p.141). The aim is to remove as much fluid as possible using an IV cannula or suprapubic catheter. Patients often feel better after the removal of as little as 2L.

Clamping the tube to reduce the drainage rate is generally unnecessary, particularly for volumes <5L. The drain should be removed after 6h, or sooner if drainage stops. Unlike ascites secondary to liver disease, hypotension is rarely a problem in paracentesis of malignancy-related ascites.[50] There is no need for IV hydration ± IV albumin.

Paracentesis can be repeated if diuretics do not prevent re-accumulation. If paracentesis has proved difficult in the past, ultrasound guidance is advisable.

Occasionally, patients living in far-distant places are treated with a semi-permanent intra-abdominal catheter.[51] One centre uses a central venous catheter, inserted into the abdomen.

Shunts
Various venous shunting procedures have been used, particularly in patients with troublesome non-malignant ascites:

● peritoneosubclavian (a valved catheter tunneled SC to the subclavian vein)
● peritoneosaphenous (proximal part of vein rotated up and anastomosed to the posterior wall of the inguinal canal).[52]

Such procedures are a potential option in a patient who is relatively well but cannot tolerate diuretic therapy. However, given the poor prognosis of most cancer patients with symptomatic ascites, shunts have little place in the management of malignant ascites. Further, in malignant ascites, peritoneo-subclavian shunts tend to block after a few weeks.[53]

Diuretics

Spironolactone is the key to success because it antagonises aldosterone (Table 4.5). Many patients are controlled on spironolactone 300mg o.d. or less.[54,55] A loop diuretic is not always necessary. The dose of the loop diuretic should be reduced or discontinued once a satisfactory result is achieved.

Failure with spironolactone generally relates to:

- gastric intolerance (less likely if given in divided dosage, i.e. t.d.s.–q.d.s.)
- too small a dose of spironolactone
- failure to use a loop diuretic concurrently in resistant cases.

Table 4.5   Diuretic treatment of malignant ascites

| | Spironolactone | Loop diuretic | |
		Furosemide or	Bumetanide
Day 1	100–200mg o.d.	–	–
Day 7	200–300mg o.d.	40mg	1mg
Day 14	200mg b.d.	80mg	2mg

Hypercalcaemia

Hypercalcaemia may cause many non-specific symptoms, e.g. dry mouth, thirst, anorexia, nausea and vomiting, constipation, frequency (polyuria), lethargy, weakness, depression. Most patients who develop hypercalcaemia have disseminated disease, and 80% die within 1 year.[56]

Incidence

All malignant disease 10–20%; up to 50% in breast cancer and myeloma. Common in squamous lung, head and neck, kidney and cervix uteri cancers. Uncommon in small cell lung, gastric, large bowel and prostate cancers.

Hypercalcaemia is mostly a paraneoplastic phenomenon.[56] Although >80% of patients with cancer-related hypercalcaemia have skeletal metastases, the extent of the disease does not correlate with the degree of hypercalcaemia.

Diagnosis is based on a high level of clinical suspicion and confirmed by blood tests, 'correcting' for hypo-albuminaemia.

Management

Stop and think! Are you justified in treating a potentially fatal complication in a moribund patient?

The following criteria jointly justify the correction of hypercalcaemia:

- corrected plasma calcium concentration of >2.8mmol/L
- symptoms attributable to hypercalcaemia
- first episode or long interval since previous one
- previous good quality of life (in the patient's opinion)
- medical expectation that treatment will achieve a durable effect (based on the results of previous treatment)
- patient willing to undergo IV therapy and requisite blood tests.

Bisphosphonates

Bisphosphonates act by inhibiting osteoclasts. Rehydrate with IV normal saline, e.g. 3L/24h, and give a bisphosphonate. Hitherto, pamidronate has been widely used:

- give 30–90mg IV, depending on plasma calcium concentration (*see* manufacturer's recommendations)
- infusion rate should not exceed 60mg/h *(20mg/h if moderate to severe renal impairment)*
- concentration should not exceed 60mg/250ml
- repeat after 1 week if the initial response inadequate
- repeat every 3–4 weeks according to plasma calcium concentration.[57]

Zoledronic acid is likely to supersede pamidronate.[58]

Spinal cord compression

Spinal cord compression occurs in 3–5% of patients with advanced cancer. Cancers of the breast, bronchus and prostate account for >60%.[59] Most occur in the thorax. There is compression at more than one level in 20%. Below the level of L2 vertebra, compression is of the cauda equina (i.e. peripheral nerves) and not the spinal cord.

Most instances of cord compression are caused by vertebral collapse or, much less commonly, by an extravertebral tumour extending through an intervertebral foramen into the epidural space (e.g. lymphoma).

Clinical features

- pain   >90%
- weakness   >75%
- sensory level   >50%
- sphincter dysfunction   >40%.

The patient may be unaware of sensory loss until examined, particularly if this is confined to the sacrum or perineum. Pain often predates other symptoms and signs of cord compression by several weeks or months. Pain may be caused by:

- vertebral metastasis
- root compression (radicular pain)
- cord compression (funicular pain)
- muscle spasm.

Radicular and funicular pains are often exacerbated by neck flexion or straight leg raising, and by coughing, sneezing or straining. Funicular pain is generally less sharp than radicular pain, has a more diffuse distribution (like a cuff or garter around the thighs, knees or calves), and is sometimes described as a cold unpleasant sensation.

Evaluation

- history and clinical findings
- a plain radiograph shows vertebral metastasis and/or collapse at the appropriate level in 80%; a bone scan does not often yield additional information
- MRI is the investigation of choice; CT with myelography may be helpful if MRI is not available.

Management

Although often insidious in onset, spinal cord compression should be treated as an emergency:

- dexamethasone, the dose used varies greatly;[59] consider 16–32mg PO daily for 1 week, and then reduce the dose progressively over 2–3 weeks
- radiation therapy, concurrently

- decompressive surgery, if there is
    deterioration despite radiotherapy and dexamethasone
    a solitary vertebral metastasis
    doubt about the diagnosis.

Patients with paraparesis do better than those who are totally paraplegic. Loss of sphincter function is a bad prognostic sign. Dexamethasone may be unnecessary in patients who are still ambulant at the time of diagnosis.[59]

If the cord compression is of rapid onset (1–2 days), the most likely cause is infarction of the spinal cord as a consequence of spinal artery thrombosis secondary to compression/distortion by malignant disease. This does not respond to treatment.

Lymphoedema

Lymphoedema is tissue swelling resulting from lymph drainage failure when capillary filtration is normal. Lymphoedema is a protein-rich oedema and is associated with chronic inflammation and fibrosis. It can occur in any part of the body but generally affects one or more limbs ± the adjacent trunk.[60,61] If left untreated, lymphoedema may become a gross and debilitating condition. Acute inflammation and trauma cause a rapid increase in swelling.

In the UK, cancer and cancer treatment account for most cases of lymphoedema. A combination of factors increases the risk:

- axillary or groin surgery
- postoperative infection
- radiotherapy
- lymph node metastases, e.g. axillary, groin, intrapelvic, retroperitoneal.

Clinical features

Symptoms include:

- tightness
- heaviness
- a bursting feeling if there is an acute exacerbation
- pain caused by
    shoulder strain (because of the weight of the arm)
    inflammation
    brachial or lumbosacral plexopathy
- impaired function/mobility

- psychosocial distress
  altered body image
  problems in obtaining well-fitting clothes or shoes.

The impact on the patient psychosocially is not always obvious. Specific enquiry is needed to elicit the extent of the patient's distress.

Unlike other types of oedema, chronic lymphoedema results in changes in the skin and subcutis. Signs include:

- persistent swelling of part or all of the limb which in time becomes non-pitting as a result of interstitial fibrosis and which does not decrease with elevation overnight
- increased tissue turgor
- Stemmer's sign (the inability to pick up a fold of skin at the base of the second toe); the absence of this sign does not necessarily exclude more proximal lymphoedema
- distorted limb shape
- lymphangiomas (dilated skin lymphatics which look like blisters)
- deep skin creases associated with cutaneous fibrosis
- hyperkeratosis (a build-up of surface keratin resulting in a warty scaly skin)
- papillomatosis (a cobblestone effect caused by dilated skin lymphatics surrounded by fibrosis)
- acute inflammatory episodes (*see* p.148)
- lymphorrhoea (leakage of lymph).

Hyperkeratosis and papillomatosis are seen mainly in lymphoedema of the leg. Lymphorrhoea is more common in lymphovenous stasis, inferior vena caval obstruction and chronic congestive cardiac failure. Ulceration is uncommon unless there is associated venous or arterial disease.

When the trunk is involved:

- the subcutis feels thickened on palpation
- when a fold of skin is pinched up simultaneously on both sides of the trunk, the skin is more difficult to grip on the affected side
- underwear leaves deeper markings on the affected side
- in unilateral leg lymphoedema, the ipsilateral buttock is bigger when examined with the patient standing
- in females, there may be genital wetness from leaking lymphangiomas.

Radiotherapy also causes subcutaneous thickening but it is qualitatively different from that in lymphoedema, i.e. it is firmer and completely non-pitting. Because muscle activity is essential to maintain both venous and lymph return from dependent limbs, lymphatic failure is also inevitable in immobile patients who sit for many hours day after day and have little or no exercise ('armchair legs'). The extra load placed on the lymphatics as a result of venous incompetence also leads to lymphatic failure. Thus, patients with chronic venous leg ulcers and swelling have a combination of venous oedema and lymphatic failure, often called lymphovenous stasis.

Management

In advanced cancer it is generally not possible to reduce the size of a lymph-oedematous limb. Emphasis should be placed on preventing deterioration and relieving discomfort.[61]

Skin care
Wash and moisturise daily, e.g. with aqueous cream. This is often best done at bedtime. Some patients benefit from initial treatment with 50/50 liquid paraffin in white soft paraffin. Give advice about avoiding trauma, thereby reducing the likelihood of infection (Box 4.P). Acute inflammatory episodes need prompt treatment with antibiotics and, if there is constitutional upset, with bed rest (Box 4.Q).

Massage
Massage is used to move lymph from the initial (non-contractile) lymphatics into the deeper muscular (contractile) collecting lymphatics.[60] All lymphoedema patients benefit from massage. Massage is the only way of clearing oedema from the trunk. Clearing the trunk increases drainage from the limb. Relatives can be taught to massage the skin. Areas affected by cutaneous cancer should not be massaged.

Compression
International standard graduation compression garments class 1–3, Shaped Tubigrip or light support bandaging (e.g. Setopress) applied daily with soft padding.[60]

Exercise
Encourage normal use or gentle active or passive movements.[60] If flaccid, use a broad arm sling when standing. Support the heavy limb when resting.

Patients must wear bandaging or a compression garment during exercise. This enhances the effect of muscle contraction on lymph flow.

Box 4.P   Written information for patients about skin care[62]

General information
If an arm is swollen, protect hands when washing up or gardening.
If a leg is swollen, wear protective footwear at all times. Do not walk in bare feet.
Wear a thimble when sewing.
Dry well between digits after bathing to protect from fungal infections.
Keep the skin supple by applying oil or bland cream.
Take care when cutting toe or finger nails; use clippers rather than scissors.
Treat any cuts or grazes promptly by washing and applying antiseptic, e.g. Savlon, TCP.
Notify your general practitioner immediately if the limb becomes hot or more swollen.
Use an electric razor to reduce the risk of cutting the skin.

Other important points about the swollen limb:
    do not have blood taken from it
    do not have injections into it
    do not allow your blood pressure to be taken on it.

Summer advice
Avoid insect bites; use repellent sprays.
Treat bites with antiseptics and/or antihistamines.
Protect the swollen limb from the sun:
    sit in the shade when possible
    use a high-factor sun block, e.g. 15–30.
Equipment to take on holiday:
    emollient
    high-factor sun block
    insect repellents/sprays
    antihistamine tablets
    antiseptic solutions.
If you have had recurrent infections, take antibiotics with you when you go on holidays in case of need.

Other
● a diuretic should be used if the swelling developed or worsened after the prescription of a NSAID or a corticosteroid, or if there is a venous component; otherwise, do *not* prescribe
● a pneumatic intermittent compression pump is helpful in shifting venous and hypo-albuminaemic oedemas; may also speed up the rate of initial improvement in patients with combined lymphovenous oedema.

Box 4.Q   Management of acute inflammatory episodes

In lymphoedema, acute inflammatory episodes (AIE), often called cellulitis, are common. AIE are frequently associated with fever, flu-like symptoms or even greater constitutional upset (e.g. nausea and vomiting). In AIE it is often difficult to isolate the pathogen responsible. However, Streptococcus is the mostly likely infective agent.

Evaluation

1 *Clinical features:*
- mild – pain, increased swelling, erythema (well-defined *or* blotchy)
- severe – extensive erythema with well-defined margins, increased swelling, blistering and weeping skin; often accompanied by fever, nausea and vomiting, pain and, when the leg is affected, difficulty in walking.

2 *Diagnosis* is based on pattern recognition and clinical judgement. The following information should be solicited:
- present history – date of onset, precipitating factor (e.g. insect bite or trauma), treatment received to date
- past history – details of previous AIE, precipitating factors, antibiotics taken
- examination – include the sites of lymphatic drainage to and from the inflamed area.

Antibiotics

3 All AIE should be treated promptly with antibiotics to prevent increased morbidity associated with increased swelling and accelerated fibrosis. In the UK, there is no standard regimen for AIE. The following is current practice in the Lymphoedema Service at Sir Michael Sobell House.

4 *No systemic upset:*

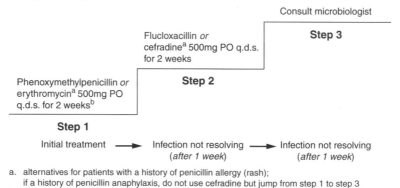

a. alternatives for patients with a history of penicillin allergy (rash);
    if a history of penicillin anaphylaxis, do not use cefradine but jump from step 1 to step 3
b. some centres use co-amoxiclav 625mg t.d.s. instead. This is active against both
    Streptococci and *Staphylococci* but causes more rashes and diarrhoea, and is more
    expensive.

5 *Systemic upset:* bed rest is crucial and may necessitate inpatient admission. Blood cultures, aspirates of bullae and surface swabs (if the skin is broken) should be taken to guide treatment in case the infection does not resolve.

continued

Meanwhile, prescribe IV antibiotics for 1 week followed by antibiotics PO for 1 week, i.e. 2 weeks in total.
Week 1:

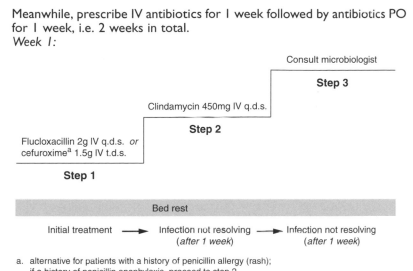

a. alternative for patients with a history of penicillin allergy (rash);
   if a history of penicillin anaphylaxis, proceed to step 2

Week 2: if the infection is resolving, continue with PO medication for a second week:
- flucloxacillin injections are replaced by capsules 500mg PO q.d.s.
- cefuroxime injections are replaced by cefradine 1g PO b.d.
- clindamycin injections are replaced by capsules 300mg PO q.d.s.

6 *Antibiotic prophylaxis:* if an AIE recurs within a year, prescribe phenoxy-methylpenicillin *500mg o.d. for one year* or cefradine if a history of penicillin rash. If a history of penicillin anaphylaxis, prescribe clindamycin 150mg o.d. instead.

General

7 Remember:
- AIE are painful; analgesics should be prescribed regularly and p.r.n.
- compression garments should not be worn until limb is comfortable
- daily skin hygiene should be continued; washing and gentle drying
- emollients should not be used in the affected area if the skin is weeping or there is an open wound
- the affected limb should be elevated in a comfortable position, supported on pillows.

8 Patients should be educated about:
- why they are susceptible to AIE, i.e. skin less robust, stagnant fluid, reduced immunity
- the consequence of AIE, i.e. increased swelling, more fibrosis, reduced response to treatment
- the importance of daily skin care, i.e. to improve and maintain the integrity of the skin
- reducing risk, e.g. protect hands when gardening, cleanse cuts, treat fungal infections
- prophylaxis with antibiotics.

Pruritus

Pruritus (itch) is a dominant symptom of skin disease and also occurs in some systemic diseases, notably cholestasis, chronic renal failure (uraemia) and malignant disease. Dry skin (xerosis) and wet macerated skin are both causes of pruritus.

Although itch of cutaneous origin shares a common neural pathway with pain, the afferent C-fibres subserving this type of itch are a functionally distinct subset which respond to histamine, acetylcholine and other pruritogens, but which are insensitive to mechanical stimuli.[63] Histamine is the main mediator for itch in insect bite reactions and in most forms of urticaria, and in these circumstances the itch responds well to H_1-antihistamines. However, in most dermatoses and in systemic disease, low-sedative H_1-antihistamines are ineffective. In these circumstances, any benefit from a sedative H_1-antihistamine (e.g. chlorphenamine, diphenhydramine) is the result of a non-specific sedative action.[64,65]

General management

Virtually all patients with advanced cancer and pruritus have a dry skin, even when there is a definite endogenous cause for the pruritus. Correcting skin dryness should therefore precede any specific measures:

- discontinue use of soap
- use emulsifying ointment or aqueous cream as a soap substitute, or add Oilatum to bath water
- avoid hot baths
- dry skin gently by patting with soft towel
- aqueous cream or alternative emollient ('moisturiser') applied to the skin after a bath or shower and each evening
- avoid overheating and sweating; this can be a particular problem at night if a winter duvet is used in the summer or with nocturnal central heating
- discourage scratching; keep nails cut short; allow gentle rubbing.

Some patients may benefit from a night sedative to reduce night-time scratching and improve sleep.

When pruritus is associated with skin maceration, the skin needs to be dried and protected from excessive moisture:

- assist evaporation by applying surgical spirit
- use a hair dryer on a cool setting
- apply a wet compress t.d.s. and allow it to dry out completely
- if infected, use an antifungal solution, e.g. clotrimazole 1%
- if very inflamed, use 1% hydrocortisone solution for 2–3 days.

Generally, do not apply adsorbent powders, e.g. starch, talc, zinc oxide, because any excess will form a hard abrasive coating on the skin.

Topical antipruritics for use with itchy skin rashes and insect bites include:

- aqueous cream plus 1–2% menthol
- oily calamine lotion p.r.n.; contains 0.5% phenol but can enhance to 1%
- antihistamine creams.

The topical use of antihistamine creams should be limited to a few days in situations where histamine is involved, e.g. an acute drug rash. A systemic H_1-antihistamine is preferrable because prolonged topical use may lead to contact dermatitis. Contact dermatitis should be treated with 1% hydrocortisone cream until the inflammation has settled.

Specific management

Opioid antagonists relieve pruritus caused by spinal opioids, cholestasis and, possibly, uraemia.[66] Itch caused by spinal opioids (but not cholestasis and uraemia) is relieved by ondansetron.[67] Other drug treatments for pruritus include:

- rifampicin, colestyramine and 17α-alkyl androgens in cholestasis (Figure 4.8)
- cimetidine and corticosteriods in Hodgkin's lymphoma (Figure 4.9)
- paroxetine if paraneoplastic (Figure 4.10)
- indometacin in some HIV+ patients[66]
- thalidomide in uraemia.[68]

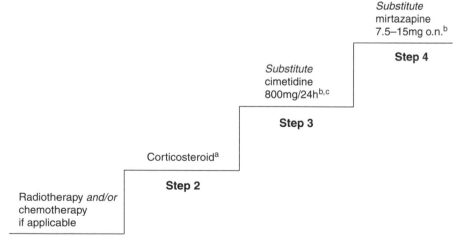

Substitute or add
colestyramine
4g × 2 o.d.– b.d.[c]

Step 4

Substitute
rifampicin
75mg o.d.–150mg b.d.

Step 3

Naltrexone
12.5–250mg o.d.[a]
or 17α-alkyl androgen[b]

Step 2

Stenting of
common bile duct

Step 1

Figure 4.8   Treatment ladder for itch in cholestasis (*see* text for references).
a. contra-indicated in patients needing opioids for pain relief
b. e.g. methyltestosterone 25mg SL o.d. (not available in UK), danazol 200mg o.d.–t.d.s.
c. *not* of benefit in complete large duct biliary obstruction.

Substitute
mirtazapine
7.5–15mg o.n.[b]

Step 4

Substitute
cimetidine
800mg/24h[b,c]

Step 3

Corticosteroid[a]

Step 2

Radiotherapy *and/or*
chemotherapy
if applicable

Step 1

Figure 4.9   Treatment ladder for itch in Hodgkin's lymphoma (*see* text for references).
a. e.g. prednisolone 30–60mg o.d. or dexamethasone 4–8mg o.d. initially
b. recommendation based on case reports
c. alternative H_2-receptor antagonists probably equally effective.

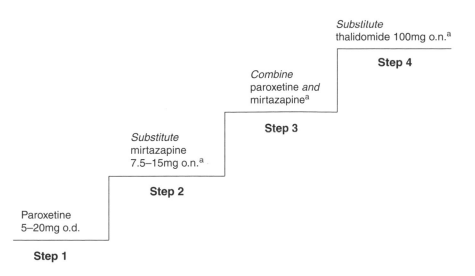

Figure 4.10   Treatment ladder for paraneoplastic itch (see text for references). a. recommendation based on case reports.

Ultraviolet B therapy, particularly narrow-band UVB, may be superior to drug treatment for uraemic pruritus.[69] If the remedies specified fail, paroxetine or mirtazapine should be considered.[66]

Secondary mental disorders

These are mental disorders which are secondary to organic disease or related to chemical substances (drugs, alcohol) or both (synonym: organic mental disorders). All types of secondary mental disorders are seen in patients with advanced cancer (Box 4.R).

Box 4.R Secondary mental disorders	
Delirium	Personality disorder
Dementia	Intoxication
Amnestic disorder	Withdrawal state
Anxiety disorder	Psychosis
Mood disorder	

Delirium (synonyms: acute brain syndrome, acute confusion), dementia (synonym: chronic brain syndrome) and amnestic disorder are all characterised by cognitive impairment. The word confusion is often used of all three conditions. Note that:

- sometimes dementia is compounded by delirium
- dementia is not generally associated with drowsiness
- some patients with cancer appear to develop dementia rapidly and this may cause difficulty in diagnosis (Box 4.S).

Box 4.S Comparison of global cognitive impairment disorders

Delirium		**Dementia**	
Acute		Chronic	
Often remitting and reversible		Usually progressive and irreversible	
Mental clouding		Brain damage	
(*information not taken in*)		(*information not retained*)	

+	Poor concentration	+
+	Impaired short-term memory	+
+	Disorientation	+
+	Living in the past	+
+	Misinterpretations	+
++	Hallucinations	+
+	Delusions	+

Delirium	**Dementia**
Speech rambling and incoherent	Speech stereotyped and limited
Often diurnal variation	Constant (in later stages)
Often aware and anxious	Unaware and unconcerned (in later stages)

Patients with cognitive impairment disorders (confusion) have identifiable cognitive defects if tested formally using, for example, the Mini-Mental State Examination. Patients manifesting the following are sometimes misdiagnosed as confused:

- not taking in what is said
    deaf
    anxious
    too ill to concentrate

- muddled speech
    poor concentration
    nominal dysphasia.

It is also important to identify hypnagogic (going to sleep) and hypnopompic (waking up) hallucinations as these are normal phenomena, although more common in ill patients receiving sedative drugs.

Causes

Dementia is usually caused by Alzheimer's disease, Lewy body disease or cerebral atherosclerosis.[70] Other causes of other secondary mental disorders are:

- drugs
- biochemical derangement
- organ failure
- brain tumours
- paraneoplastic.

Delirium

Delirium (synonym: acute confusional state) is the result of mental clouding. This leads to a disturbance of comprehension and bewilderment. Manifestations include:

- poor concentration
- impairment of short-term memory
- disorientation
- misinterpretations
- paranoid delusions
- hallucinations
- rambling incoherent speech
- agitation
- noisy/aggressive behaviour.

There may be associated drowsiness. Psychomotor activity may be increased or decreased. Increased activity may be associated with overactivity of the autonomic nervous system manifesting as facial flushing, dilated pupils, injected conjunctivae, tachycardia and sweating.

Management

Correct the correctable
Delirium is generally a reversible condition and an underlying cause should be sought and appropriately treated (Box 4.T).[71,72] Common causes are infection and medication, e.g. psychotropics, opioids, corticosteroids. In more than 1/2 of patients with advanced cancer and delirium the cause may not be identified.[73]

Box 4.T Precipitating factors for delirium in advanced cancer

Change of environment	Biochemical disturbances
Unfamiliar excessive stimuli	hypercalcaemia
too hot	hyponatraemia
too cold	Drug-induced
wet bed	opioids
crumbs in bed	antimuscarinics
creases in sheets	corticosteroids
General deterioration	chemotherapy agents, e.g. cisplatin, 5-FU,
Fatigue	ifosfamide, methotrexate
Anxiety	immunomodulators, e.g. interferon,
Depression	interleukin
Pain	Withdrawal state
Faecal impaction	alcohol
Urinary retention	nicotine
Infection	psychotropic drugs
Dehydration	Thiamine deficiency
Brain tumour(s)	

If nicotine withdrawal is suspected, encourage smoking or administer a medicinal nicotine product:

● Nicorette nasal spray, containing nicotine 500microgram/metered spray
● TD nicotine patches, 11mg and 22mg in 24h.

The cost of TD patches is not covered by the NHS in the UK.

Non-drug treatment
An attempt should be made to help the patient to express their distress. Hallucinations, nightmares and misinterpretations often reflect the patient's

fears and anxieties. Their content should be explored with the patient. In addition:

- keep calm and avoid confrontation
- respond to the patient's comments
- clarify perceptions, and validate those which are accurate
- explain what is happening and why
- state what can be done to help
- repeat important and helpful information
- when indicated, recommend some tablets or an injection 'to help settle things down so that you can relax and rest for a few hours'
- stress to both the patient and the family that delirium is not madness, and that they can expect lucid intervals
- continue to treat the patient with courtesy and respect
- restraints should never be used
- bed rails should be avoided, they can be dangerous
- patient should be allowed to walk about accompanied
- allay fear and suspicion, and reduce misinterpretations by
  use of night light
  not changing the position of the patient's bed
  explaining every procedure and event in detail
  the presence of a family member or close friend.

In severe delirium, the doctor should acknowledge and accept the patient's distress, e.g. 'I can see that you are very upset', and invite the patient to return to his room and/or bed so that they can discuss things further. The presence of a close relative or friend, continuity of professional carers and a single room to minimise external visual and auditory stimulation may all help to provide a safe environment.[74]

Drug treatment

Generally use drugs only if symptoms are marked, persistent and cause distress to the patient and/or family. Review sooner rather than later if a sedative drug is prescribed because symptoms may be exacerbated. Consider:

- reduction in medication
- oxygen if cyanosed
- dexamethasone if cerebral tumour (see p.164)
- haloperidol 1.5–5mg PO or SC if agitated, hallucinated or paranoid.

The initial dose of haloperidol depends on previous medication, weight, age and severity of symptoms. Subsequent doses depend on the initial response. Daily or b.d. maintenance doses are generally adequate; sometimes more frequent administration is necessary.

An atypical antipsychotic, e.g. olanzapine, risperidone, can be used instead, although in the UK injections are not yet available.

Terminal agitation

This is often associated with delirium and may need haloperidol 10–30mg/24h and/or midazolam 10–60mg/24h by CSCI to control it.

In a few patients such measures are inadequate, and they continue to be agitated. Those 'at risk' include war veterans, holocaust survivors, and those who have been abused or tortured. If bitter repressed memories have not been brought to the surface and dealt with in the past, or in the weeks or months before death, they will almost certainly 'erupt' when a person develops delirium.[75]

In such circumstances, if imminently dying, it may become necessary to sedate someone so that they are unconscious until death comes.[76,77] A sedative antipsychotic, such as levomepromazine (methotrimeprazine) 25–50mg stat and 50–200mg/24h (or more), should be substituted for haloperidol, and given together with midazolam. Alternatively, SC phenobarbital 100–200mg stat and 800–1600mg/24h could be given instead of both haloperidol and midazolam.

References

1 Moertel C *et al.* (1974) Corticosteroid therapy for preterminal gastrointestinal cancer. *Cancer.* **33:** 1607–1609.
2 Bruera E *et al.* (1985) Action of oral methylprednisolone in terminal cancer patients: a prospective randomized double-blind study. *Cancer Treatment Reports.* **69:** 751–754.
3 Bruera E *et al.* (1998) Effectiveness of megestrol acetate in patients with advanced cancer: a randomized, double-blind, crossover study. *Cancer Prevention Control.* **2:** 74–78.
4 Westman G *et al.* (1999) Megestrol acetate in advanced, progressive, hormone-insensitive cancer. Effects on the quality of life: a placebo-controlled, randomised, multicentre trial. *European Journal of Cancer.* **35:** 586–595.
5 Bruera E and Higginson I (1996) *Cachexia-Anorexia in Cancer Patients.* Oxford University Press, Oxford.
6 Puccio M and Nathanson L (1997) The cancer cachexia syndrome. *Seminars in Oncology.* **24:** 277–287.
7 Hussey H and Tisdale M (1999) Effect of cachectic factor on carbohydrate metabolism and attenuation by eicosapentaenoic acid. *British Journal of Cancer.* **80:** 1231–1235.
8 Jaskowiak N and Alexander H (1997) The pathophysiology of cancer cachexia. In: D Doyle *et al.* (eds) *Oxford Textbook of Palliative Medicine.* Oxford University Press, Oxford, pp 534–548.
9 Preston T *et al.* (1995) Effect of ibuprofen on the acute-phase response and protein metabolism in patients with cancer and weight loss. *British Journal of Surgery.* **82:** 229–234.
10 McMillan D *et al.* (1998) Longitudinal study of body cell mass depletion and the inflammatory response in cancer patients. *Nutrition and Cancer.* **31:** 101–105.

11 Barber M *et al.* (1998) Current controversies in cancer. Should cancer patients with incurable disease receive parenteral or enteral nutritional support? *European Journal of Cancer.* **34:** 279–285.

12 Bruera E and MacDonald N (1988) Nutrition in cancer patients: an update and review of our experience. *Journal of Pain and Symptom Management.* **3:** 133–140.

13 Gagnon B and Bruera E (1998) A review of the drug treatment of cachexia associated with cancer. *Drugs.* **55:** 675–688.

14 Strang P (1997) The effect of megestrol acetate on anorexia, weight loss and cachexia in cancer and AIDS patients (review). *Anticancer Research.* **17:** 657–662.

15 Vadell C *et al.* (1998) Anticachectic efficacy of megestrol acetate at different doses and versus placebo in patients with neoplastic cachexia. *American Journal of Clinical Oncology.* **21:** 347–351.

16 McMillan D *et al.* (1997) A pilot study of megestrol acetate and ibuprofen in the treatment of cachexia in gastrointestinal cancer patients. *British Journal of Cancer.* **76:** 788–790.

17 Twycross RG and Lack SA (1986) *Control of Alimentary Symptoms in Far Advanced Cancer.* Churchill Livingstone, Edinburgh.

18 Nelson K *et al.* (1993) Assessment of upper gastrointestinal motility in the cancer-associated dyspepsia syndrome (CADS). *Journal of Palliative Care.* **9:** 27–31.

19 Yeomans N *et al.* (1998) A comparison of omeprazole with ranitidine for ulcers associated with nonsteroidal anti-inflammatory drugs. Acid suppression trial. *New England Journal of Medicine.* **338:** 719–726.

20 Hawkey C *et al.* (1998) Omeprazole compared with misoprostol for ulcers associated with nonsteroidal anti-inflammatory drugs. *New England Journal of Medicine.* **338:** 727–734.

21 Lichter I (1993) Results of antiemetic management in terminal illness. *Journal of Palliative Care.* **9:** 19–21.

22 Tjeerdsma II *et al.* (1993) Voluntary suppression of defecation delays gastric emptying. *Digestive Diseases and Sciences.* **38:** 832–836.

23 Schuurkes JAJ *et al.* (1986) Stimulation of gastroduodenal motor activity: dopaminergic and cholinergic modulation. *Drug Development Research.* **8:** 233–241.

24 De-Conno F *et al.* (1991) Continuous subcutaneous infusion of hyoscine butylbromide reduces secretion in patients with gastrointestinal obstruction. *Journal of Pain and Symptom Management.* **6:** 484–486.

25 Mercadante S *et al.* (2000) Comparison of octreotide and hyoscine butylbromide in controlling gastrointestinal symptoms due to malignant inoperable bowel obstruction. *Supportive Care in Cancer.* **8:** 188–191.

26 Harris A and Cantwell B (1986) Mechanisms and treatment of cytotoxic-induced nausea and vomiting. In: C Davis *et al.* (eds) *Nausea and Vomiting: mechanisms and treatment.* Springer-Verlag, Berlin, pp 78–93.

27 Krebs H and Goplerud D (1987) Mechanical intestinal obstruction in patients with gynecologic disease: a review of 368 patients. *American Journal of Obstetrics and Gynecology.* **157:** 577–583.

28 Ripamonti C *et al.* (2001) Clinical-practice recommendations for the management of bowel obstruction in patients with end-stage cancer. *Supportive Care in Cancer.* **9:** 223–233.

29 Feuer D and Broadley K (1999) Systematic review and meta-analysis of corticosteroids for the resolution of malignant bowel obstruction in advanced gynaecological and gastrointestinal cancers. *Annals of Oncology.* **10:** 1035–1041.

30 Laval G *et al.* (2000) The use of steroids in the management of inoperable intestinal obstruction in terminal cancer patients: do they remove the obstruction? *Palliative Medicine.* **14:** 3–10.

31 Ashby M *et al.* (1991) Percutaneous gastrostomy as a venting procedure in palliative care. *Palliative Medicine.* **5:** 147–150.

32 Reuben DB and Mor V (1986) Dyspnoea in terminally ill cancer patients. *Chest.* **89:** 234–236.

33 O'Driscoll M *et al.* (1999) The experience of breathlessness in lung cancer. *European Journal of Cancer Care.* **8:** 37–43.

34 Davis C (1997) Breathlessness, cough, and other respiratory problems. *British Medical Journal.* **315:** 931–934.
35 Dudgeon D and Lertzman M (1999) Dyspnea in the advanced cancer patient. *Journal of Pain and Symptom Management.* **16:** 212–219.
36 Bredin M *et al.* (1999) Multicentre randomized controlled trial of nursing intervention for breathlessness in patients with lung cancer. *British Medical Journal.* **318:** 901–904.
37 Heijden Hvd *et al.* (1996) Pharmacotherapy of respiratory muscles in chronic obstructive pulmonary disease. *Respiratory Medicine.* **90:** 513–522.
38 Davis C *et al.* (1996) Single dose randomized controlled trial of nebulized morphine in patients with cancer related breathlessness. *Palliative Medicine.* **10:** 64–65.
39 Marshall J (1997) Panic disorder: a treatment update. *Journal of Clinical Psychiatry.* **58:** 36–42.
40 Hughes A *et al.* (2000) Audit of three antimuscarinic drugs for managing retained secretions. *Palliative Medicine.* **14:** 221–222.
41 Bennett M *et al.* (2002) Using anti-muscarinic drugs in the management of death rattle: evidence based guidelines for palliative care. *Palliative Medicine.* **16:** 369–374.
42 Wildiers H and Menten J (2002) Death rattle: prevalence, prevention and treatment. *Journal of Pain and Symptom Management.* **23:** 310–317.
43 De-Ruysscher D *et al.* (1996) Treatment of intractable hiccup in a terminal cancer patient with nebulized saline. *Palliative Medicine.* **10:** 166–167.
44 Guelaud C *et al.* (1995) Baclofen therapy for chronic hiccup. *European Respiratory Journal.* **8:** 235–237.
45 Brigham B and Bolin T (1992) High dose nifedipine and fludrocortisone for intractable hiccups. *Medical Journal of Australia.* **157:** 70.
46 Ives TJ *et al.* (1985) Treatment of intractable hiccups with intramuscular haloperidol. *American Journal of Psychiatry.* **142:** 1368–1369.
47 Jacobson P *et al.* (1981) Treatment of intractable hiccups with valproic acid. *Neurology.* **31:** 1458–1460.
48 Wilcock A and Twycross R (1996) Case report: midazolam for intractable hiccup. *Journal of Pain and Symptom Management.* **12:** 59–61.
49 Twycross R and Wilcock A (2001) *Symptom Management in Advanced Cancer* (3e). Radcliffe Medical Press, Oxford, pp 294–295.
50 Stephenson J and Gilbert J (2002) The development of clinical guidelines on paracentesis for ascites related to malignancy. *Palliative Medicine.* **16:** 213–218.
51 Iyengar T and Herzog T (2002) Management of symptomatic ascites in recurrent ovarian cancer patients using an intra-abdominal semi-permanent catheter. *American Journal of Hospice and Palliative Care.* **19:** 35–38.
52 Deen K *et al.* (2001) Saphenoperitoneal anastomosis for resistant ascites in patients with cirrhosis. *American Journal of Surgery.* **181:** 145–148.
53 Soderlund C (1986) Denver peritoneovenous shunting for malignant or cirrhotic ascites. A prospective consecutive series. *Scandinavian Journal of Gastroenterology.* **21:** 1167–1172.
54 Fogel M *et al.* (1981) Diuresis in the ascitic patient: a randomized controlled trial of three regimens. *Journal of Clinical Gastroenterology.* **3:** 73–80.
55 Greenway B *et al.* (1982) Control of malignant ascites with spironolactone. *British Journal of Surgery.* **69:** 441–442.
56 Bower M *et al.* (1997) Endocrine and metabolic complications of advanced cancer. In: D Doyle *et al.* (eds) *Oxford Textbook of Palliative Medicine.* Oxford University Press, Oxford, pp 709–725.
57 Twycross R *et al.* (2002) *Palliative Care Formulary* (2e). Radcliffe Medical Press, Oxford, pp 215–218.
58 Major P *et al.* (2001) Zoledronic acid is superior to pamidronate in the treatment of hypercalcaemia of malignancy. a pooled analysis of two randomized, controlled clinical trials. *Journal of Clinical Oncology.* **19:** 558–567.

59 Loblaw D and Laperriere N (1998) Emergency treatment of malignant extradural spinal cord compression: an evidence-based guideline. *Journal of Clinical Oncology.* **16:** 1613–1624.
60 Twycross R *et al.* (2000) *Lymphoedema.* Radcliffe Medical Press, Oxford.
61 Twycross R and Wilcock A (2001) *Symptom Management in Advanced Cancer* (3e). Radcliffe Medical Press, Oxford, pp 339–357.
62 Linnitt N (2000) Skin management in lymphoedema. In: R Twycross *et al.* (eds) *Lymphoedema.* Radcliffe Medical Press, Oxford, pp 118–129.
63 Schmelz M *et al.* (1997) Specific C-receptors for itch in human skin. *Journal of Neuroscience.* **17:** 8003–8008.
64 Krause L and Shuster S (1983) Mechanisms of action of antipruritic drugs. *British Medical Journal.* **287:** 1199–1200.
65 Berth-Jones J and Graham-Brown R (1989) Failure of terfenadine in relieving the pruritus of atopic dermatitis. *British Journal of Dermatology.* **121:** 635–637.
66 Twycross R *et al.* (2002) Itch: scratching more than the surface. *Quarterly Journal of Medicine.* In press.
67 Borgeat A and Stimemann H-R (1999) Ondansetron is effective to treat spinal or epidural morphine-induced pruritus. *Anesthesiology.* **90:** 432–436.
68 Silvas *et al.* (1994) Thalidomide for the treatment of uremic pruritus: a crossover randomized double-blind trial. *Nephron.* **67:** 270–2/3.
69 Szepietowski J *et al.* (2002) Ultraviolet B induces mast cell apoptosis: a hypothetical mechanism of ultraviolet B treatment for uraemic pruritus. *Medical Hypotheses.* **58:** 167–170.
70 American Psychiatric Association (1994) Dementia. *Diagnostic and Statistical Manual of Mental Disorders,* 4th edition (DSM-IV). American Psychiatric Association, New York.
71 American Psychiatric Association (1999) Practice guideline for the treatment of patients with delirium. *American Journal of Psychiatry.* **156:** 1–18.
72 Cole M (1999) Delirium: effectiveness of systematic interventions. *Dementia and Geriatric Cognitive Disorders.* **10:** 406–411.
73 Bruera E *et al.* (1992) Cognitive failure in patients with terminal cancer: A prospective study. *Journal of Pain and Symptom Management.* **7:** 192–195.
74 Macleod A (1997) The management of delirium in hospice practice. *European Journal of Palliative Care.* **4:** 116–120.
75 Stedeford A (1994) *Facing death: patients, families and professionals.* Sobell Publications, Oxford.
76 Fainsinger R *et al.* (2000) Sedation for delirium and other symptoms in terminally ill patients in Edmonton. *Journal of Palliative Care.* **16(2):** 5–10.
77 Cowan J and Walsh D (2001) Terminal sedation in palliative medicine – definition and review of the literature. *Supportive Care in Cancer.* **9:** 403–407.

PART FIVE

Drug profiles

Antacids · Corticosteroids · Benzodiazepines
Diazepam · Midazolam · Haloperidol
Antimuscarinics · Hyoscine

Antacids

Antacids neutralise gastric acid:

- sodium bicarbonate
- magnesium salts (may also cause diarrhoea)
- aluminium hydroxide (may also cause constipation)
- hydrotalcite (aluminium magnesium carbonate)
- calcium carbonate.[1]

Most proprietary preparations contain a mixture of magnesium salts and aluminium salts so as to have a neutral impact on intestinal transit.

Some antacids contain significant amounts of sodium. This may be important in patients with hypertension or cardiac failure. *Liquid Gaviscon and magnesium trisilicate mixture both contain >6mmol/10ml*, whereas Asilone contains only 0.1mmol/10ml. Regular use of sodium bicarbonate can cause sodium loading and metabolic alkalosis.

Aluminium hydroxide binds dietary phosphate. It is of benefit in patients with hyperphosphataemia in renal failure. Long-term complications of phosphate depletion and osteomalacia are not an issue in advanced cancer.

Hydrotalcite binds bile salts and is of specific benefit in patients with bile salt reflux, e.g. after certain forms of gastroduodenal surgery.

Regular use of calcium carbonate may cause hypercalcaemia, particularly if taken with sodium bicarbonate.

Special preparations

Some antacids contain additional substances for use in specific situations:

- alginic acid (in Gaviscon) prevents oesophageal reflux pain by forming an inert low density raft on the top of the acid stomach contents. Gaviscon needs both acid and air bubbles to produce the raft; it may be less effective if used with an H_2-receptor antagonist or a proton pump inhibitor (reduces acid) and/or antiflatulent (reduces air bubbles)

- dimeticone (dimethylpolysiloxane) is an antifoaming agent present in some proprietary antacids, e.g. Asilone and Maalox Plus. By facilitating belching, dimeticone eases flatulence, distension and postprandial gastric pain.

Points to remember

- *the administration of antacids should be separated from the administration of enteric-coated tablets;* direct contact between enteric-coated tablets and antacids may result in damage to the coating with consequential exposure of the stomach mucosa to the drug, and of the drug to gastric acid
- apart from sodium bicarbonate, antacids delay gastric emptying and may thereby modify drug absorption
- some proprietary preparations contain peppermint oil which masks the chalky taste of the antacid and helps belching by decreasing the tone of the lower oesophageal sphincter
- most antacid tablets feel gritty when sucked; some patients dislike this
- some proprietary preparations are fruit-flavoured, e.g. Tums (chewable tablet) and Remegel (chewing gum)
- the cheapest preparations are magnesium trisilicate BP and aluminium hydroxide gel BP given alone or as a mixture.

For optimum impact, antacids are best administered 1h after meals. This maximises contact time with gastric acid; o.n. and p.r.n. doses can also be taken. However, if acid suppression around the clock is the aim, an H_2-receptor antagonist or proton pump inhibitor should be prescribed instead.

Corticosteroids

Corticosteroids are used for many reasons in advanced cancer (Box 5.A).[2] Inclusion in the table does *not* mean that a corticosteroid is the treatment of choice in that situation.

At Sir Michael Sobell House, dexamethasone is the corticosteroid of choice. It is generally given in a single daily dose. Dexamethasone has a duration of effect of 36–54h, compared with 18–36h for prednisolone. Oral bio-availability for both drugs is about 80%.

Box 5.A Indications for corticosteroids in advanced cancer

Specific
Anti-emetic
Spinal cord compression
Nerve compression
Breathlessness
   pneumonitis (after radiotherapy)
   lymphangitis carcinomatosa
   tracheal compression/stridor
Superior vena caval obstruction
Obstruction of hollow viscus
   bronchus
   ureter
   bowel
Radiation-induced inflammation
Rectal discharge (give PR)

Pain relief
Raised intracranial pressure
Nerve compression
Spinal cord compression
Bone pain

Hormone therapy
Replacement
Anticancer

General
To improve appetite
To enhance sense of wellbeing

Dexamethasone is 7 times more potent than prednisolone. Thus, 2mg of dexamethasone is approximately equivalent to 15mg of prednisolone. In the UK, dexamethasone is available in 0.5mg and 2mg tablets, and also as an injection. Prednisolone is available in a range of sizes from 1–25mg.

The initial daily dose varies according to indication and fashion, ranging from dexamethasone 2–4mg (prednisolone 15–30mg) for anorexia to dexamethasone 16–32mg for spinal cord compression. A dose of 8–16mg is generally used for raised intracranial pressure.

Moonfacing, hyperphagia, weight gain, myopathy or diabetes mellitus may necessitate dose reduction and occasionally stopping treatment. Ankle oedema is common. Agitation, insomnia or a more florid psychiatric disturbance may be precipitated by corticosteroids, either when commencing or stopping treatment.

Apart from hydrocortisone, corticosteroids should generally be given in a single daily dose in the morning to ease compliance and to prevent insomnia. Even so, temazepam or diazepam at bedtime is sometimes needed to counter insomnia or increased anxiety.

Stopping corticosteroids

If after 7–10 days the corticosteroid fails to achieve the desired effect, it should be stopped. It is often possible to stop abruptly (Box 5.B). However, if there is uncertainty about disease or symptom resolution, withdrawal should be guided by monitoring disease activity or the symptom.

After whole-brain radiation, dexamethasone 4mg should be maintained for at least 1 week and the dose then reduced at the rate of 1mg/week.[3] In dying patients who are no longer able to swallow medication, it is generally acceptable to discontinue corticosteroids abruptly.

Box 5.B   Recommendations for withdrawing systemic corticosteroids[4]

Abrupt withdrawal
Systemic corticosteroids may be stopped abruptly in those whose disease is unlikely to relapse *and* have received treatment for <3 weeks *and* are not in the groups below.

Gradual withdrawal
Gradual withdrawal of systemic corticosteroids is advisable in patients who:
- have received more than 3 weeks' treatment.
- have received prednisolone >40mg daily or equivalent, e.g. dexamethasone 4–6mg
- have had a second dose in the evening
- are taking a short course within 1 year of stopping long-term therapy
- have other possible causes of adrenal suppression.

During corticosteroid withdrawal the dose may initially be reduced rapidly down to physiological doses (prednisolone 7.5mg daily or equivalent), and then more slowly (e.g. 1–2mg per week) to allow the adrenals to recover and to prevent a hypo-adrenal crisis (malaise, profound weakness, hypotension, etc.) The patient should be monitored during withdrawal in case of deterioration.

Benzodiazepines

Benzodiazepines are indicated for various symptoms in palliative care (Box 5.C).[5] At Sir Michael Sobell House, diazepam and midazolam are used almost exclusively (see below). Delirium is generally best treated with an antipsychotic (e.g. haloperidol, olanzapine, risperidone); benzodiazepines may well make matters worse. Delirium tremors (alcohol withdrawal) is the main exception to this rule. The use of benzodiazepines generally is limited by:

- drowsiness
- muscle flaccidity
- postural hypotension.

Not surprisingly, benzodiazepines are associated with falls in the elderly.

Box 5.C   Benzodiazepines in palliative care[5]

Night sedation
Short-acting drugs
- midazolam is not available in tablet form in the UK (halflife = 2–5h)
- zopiclone and zolpidem are alternatives available in the UK (halflives = 2–5h); they are not benzodiazepines but act on the same receptors.

Intermediate-acting drug
- temazepam 10–40mg PO o.n., occasionally 60mg, is widely used (halflife = 8–15h).

Long-acting drug
- flunitrazepam, although marketed as a night sedative (0.5–2mg), has a plasma halflife of 16–35h; it is therefore *not* recommended as a night sedative in palliative care.

Some patients with insomnia respond better to an antipsychotic drug or a sedative tricyclic antidepressant.

Anxiety and panic disorder
Intermediate-acting drugs
- oxazepam 10–15mg PO b.d.–t.d.s. (halflife = 5–15h)
- lorazepam 1–2mg PO b.d.–t.d.s. (halflife = 10–20h).

Lorazepam tablets are used SL at some centres for episodes of acute severe distress (e.g. respiratory panic attacks). For regular use, given its halflife, o.n. or b.d. administration should suffice.

Long-acting drug
- diazepam 2–20mg PO o.n. (halflife = 20–100h).

The BNF recommends t.d.s. administration but the long halflife means that o.n. will generally be as effective, and easier for the patient.

Acute psychotic agitation
In acute psychotic agitation, lorazepam 2mg PO/IM every 30min until settled is as effective as haloperidol 5mg every 30min.[6]

Muscle relaxant
- diazepam 2–10mg PO o.n., occasionally more
- baclofen is a useful non-benzodiazepine alternative, particularly if diazepam is too sedative and anxiety is not an associated problem.

Anti-epileptic
Acute treatment[7]
- clonazepam 1mg IV, injected over 30sec; repeat after 15min × 2 p.r.n.[8]
- diazepam 10mg IV, injected over 2–4min; repeat after 15min × 2 p.r.n.

continued

Box 5.C   Continued

- lorazepam 100microgram/kg IV, injected at 2mg/min[8,9]
- midazolam 10mg IV, injected over 2min; repeat after 15min × 2 p.r.n.

Chronic treatment
- clonazepam 500microgram–1mg PO o.n., rising by 500microgram every 3–5 days up to 2–4mg, occasionally more; doses above 2mg can be divided, e.g. 2mg o.n. and the rest o.m.

Myoclonus
Same choice as for seizures but lower doses:
- diazepam 5mg PO o.n.
- midazolam 5mg SC stat and 10mg/24h CSCI in moribund patients.

Alcohol withdrawal
Same choice as for seizure with dose and route dependent on severity of withdrawal syndrome.[10,11]

Diazepam

Diazepam is used mainly in the management of:

- anxiety
- insomnia
- muscle spasm
- seizures.[12]

The following should be noted:

- plasma halflife 20–100h; generally given as a single daily dose at bedtime. If the patient does not sleep at night, daytime drowsiness is more likely
- oral bio-availability is almost 100%
- occasional patients become more anxious; if this happens, change to haloperidol
- diazepam acts faster PO or PR than IM because the standard injection is oil-based; IV injection may cause thrombophlebitis
- if available, use diazepam oil-in-water emulsion (Diazemuls) for IV injection; it is less irritant.

Therapeutic guidelines

Initial dose depends on:

- patient's previous experience of diazepam and other benzodiazepines
- intensity of distress
- urgency of relief.

Typical doses for diazepam are given in Table 5.1. Repeat hourly until the desired effect is achieved, and then decide on an appropriate maintenance regimen, generally a single daily dose given at bedtime. More frequent dosing (b.d. or t.d.s.) is sometimes indicated in an agitated moribund patient to reduce the number of hours awake.

Table 5.1 Dose recommendations for diazepam

Indication	Stat and p.r.n. doses	Initial daily dose	Common range
Anxiety[a]	2–10mg PO	2–10mg PO o.n.	2–20mg PO
Muscle spasm[b] Multifocal myoclonus	5mg PO	5mg PO o.n.	2–10mg PO
Anti-epileptic[c]	10mg PR/IV	10–20mg	10–30mg

a. given as an adjunct to non-drug approaches, e.g. relaxation therapy and massage
b. if localised, consider injection of a trigger point with local anaesthetic or acupuncture
c. acute use but in the moribund can be used as a convenient substitute for long-term oral anti-epileptic therapy (also *see* midazolam below).

Rectal diazepam is useful in a crisis or if the patient is moribund:

- suppositories 10mg
- rectal solution 5–10mg in 2.5ml
- parenteral formulation inserted through a cannula.

Alternatively, lorazepam 1mg SL can be given (equivalent to diazepam 10mg).

Midazolam

SC/IV injections of midazolam are used mainly for:

- anaesthetic induction
- sedation for minor procedures
- seizure control
- agitation in patients who are imminently dying.[13]

It has also been used for intractable hiccup.[14]

The main advantage of midazolam is that it is water-soluble and miscible with most of the drugs commonly given by CSCI. When given IV, it causes less phlebitis than diazepam. In single doses:

- for sedation, midazolam is 3 times more potent than diazepam
- as an anti-epileptic, midazolam is twice as potent as diazepam.

With multiple doses, diazepam will gain in potency because of its prolonged plasma halflife, i.e. 20–100h versus 2.5h for midazolam (but about 10h when given by infusion). In renal impairment, cumulation of an active metabolite, hydroxymidazolam glucuronide, occurs and this can cause prolonged sedation.[15]

Oral bio-availability varies from 30–70% (tablets are not available in the UK).

Therapeutic guidelines

Typical doses for midazolam are shown in Table 5.2.

Table 5.2   Dose recommendations for SC midazolam

Indication	Stat and p.r.n. doses	Initial infusion rate/24h	Common range
Muscle tension/spasm Multifocal myoclonus	5mg	10mg	10–30mg
Terminal agitation Intractable hiccup	5–10mg[a]	30mg	30–60mg[b]
Anti-epileptic	10mg	30mg	30–60mg

a. for hiccup, give initial stat dose IV
b. reported upper dose range = 120mg for hiccup; 240mg for agitation.

In terminal agitation, if the patient does not settle on 30mg/24h, an anti-psychotic (e.g. haloperidol) should be introduced before further increasing the dose of midazolam.

Haloperidol

Haloperidol is a 'typical' antipsychotic; it acts through antagonism of dopamine type 2 receptors in the brain. In palliative care, haloperidol is used mainly as an:

- anti-emetic
- antipsychotic
- anxiolytic in delirium.[16]

It is also used in intractable hiccup.

The following should be noted:

- can generally be given as a single daily dose at bedtime; plasma halflife 13–35h
- oral bio-availability is 60–70%
- extrapyramidal effects are more likely at daily doses of <5mg; these do not occur predictably and an antiparkinsonian drug should not be prescribed prophylactically
- is the anxiolytic of choice if a patient is hallucinating, paranoid, or in agitated delirium.

Compared with chlorpromazine, haloperidol causes:

- less sedation
- less cardiovascular effects
- little or no antimuscarinic effects
- more extrapyramidal reactions, notably akathisia (motor restlessness).

For long-term use in schizophrenia, atypical antipsychotics (e.g. olanzapine, risperidone) are preferable to haloperidol because they cause fewer drug-induced movement disorders.[17,18] This possibly relates to the fact that, with atypical antipsychotics, dopamine type 2 receptor antagonism is balanced by serotonin ($5HT_2$)-receptor antagonism.[19]

Therapeutic guidelines

In the UK, haloperidol is available as a solution (1mg/ml, 2mg/ml), capsule (0.5mg), tablet (1.5, 5, 10, 20mg) and an injection. Typical doses for haloperidol are shown in Table 5.3. Plasma concentrations are approximately halved by concurrent use of carbamazepine.

Table 5.3   Dose recommendations for PO haloperidol

Indication	Stat and p.r.n. doses	Initial rate/24h	Common range
Anti-emetic[a]	1.5mg	1.5mg o.n.	1.5–5mg o.n.
Antipsychotic Delirium	1.5–5mg	1.5–5mg o.n.	1.5–10mg o.n.[b]

a. for chemical and toxic causes of vomiting
b. some patients need more, occasionally 20mg o.n. or 10mg b.d.

Antimuscarinics

'Dry as a bone, blind as a bat, red as a beet, hot as a hare, mad as a hatter.'

Antimuscarinics (anticholinergics) are used principally as smooth muscle antispasmodics and antisecretory drugs.[20] They comprise the natural belladonna alkaloids (atropine and hyoscine) and synthetic and semi-synthetic derivatives. The derivatives are divided into tertiary amines, e.g. dicycloverine (dicyclomine), and quaternary ammonium compounds, e.g. hyoscine *butylbromide*, glyco-pyrronium and propantheline.

The quaternary ammonium compounds are less lipid-soluble than the natural belladonna alkaloids, are less likely to cross the blood-brain barrier but are also less well absorbed from the gastro-intestinal tract. Central antimuscarinic-like effects (e.g. delirium) are therefore not a problem but peripheral antimuscarinic effects are characteristic (Box 5.D).

Box 5.D Peripheral antimuscarinic effects

Visual
Mydriasis ⎫
Loss of accommodation ⎬ blurred vision

Gastro-intestinal
Dry mouth
Heartburn
Constipation

Cardiovascular
Palpitations ⎫ also related to noradrenaline
Extrasystoles ⎬ (norepinephrine) potentiation
Arrhythmias ⎭ and a quinidine-like action

Urinary tract
Hesitancy of micturition
Retention of urine

Some other drugs used in palliative care also have antimuscarinic properties (Box 5.E). Antimuscarinic effects may be a limiting factor in their use. The concurrent use of two drugs with antimuscarinic properties should generally be avoided.

Antimuscarinics block the final common (cholinergic) pathway through which prokinetics act; *the two types of drugs should not be prescribed concurrently.*[21] Antimuscarinics relax the lower oesophageal sphincter and, if possible, should be avoided in patients with symptomatic acid reflux. Antimuscarinics should be avoided in paralytic ileus. Glaucoma may be precipitated in those at risk, particularly the elderly.

Box 5.E Drugs with antimuscarinic properties used in palliative care

Antihistamines
 chlorphenamine
  (chlorpheniramine)
 cyclizine[a]
 dimenhydrinate[a,b]
 promethazine[a,b]

Antiparkinsonians
 orphenadrine
 procyclidine

Antispasmodics
 mebeverine
 oxybutynin
 propantheline

Belladonna alkaloids
 atropine
 hyoscine

Glycopyrronium

Phenothiazines
 chlorpromazine
 levomepromazine
  (methotrimeprazine)
 prochlorperazine

Tricyclic antidepressants

---

a. these are antihistaminic anti-emetics
b. not much used in UK.

Hyoscine

Hyoscine (scopolamine) is an antimuscarinic with smooth muscle relaxant (antispasmodic) and antisecretory properties.[22] It is available as *hydrobromide* and *butylbromide* (Buscopan) salts. The latter is a quaternary salt and does not cross the blood-brain barrier. Unlike hyoscine *hydrobromide*, hyoscine *butylbromide* does not cause drowsiness nor does it have a central anti-emetic action.

The following should be noted:

- hyoscine *butylbromide* is poorly absorbed PO. By mouth it is of use only in intestinal colic
- repeated administration of hyoscine *hydrobromide* leads to cumulation and may result paradoxically in an agitated delirium. If this occurs, add diazepam or midazolam and consider changing to hyoscine *butylbromide*.

In the UK, hyoscine *butylbromide* is available as 10mg tablets and 20mg ampoules. Hyoscine *hydrobromide* is available as:

- 300microgram tablet *for sublingual use*
- 400microgram, 600microgram ampoules
- a transdermal patch delivering 1mg over 3 days.

Therapeutic guidelines

Injections of hyoscine *butylbromide* are cheaper than hyoscine *hydrobromide* and should generally be used in preference. Typical doses for hyoscine *butylbromide* are shown in Table 5.4.

Table 5.4   Dose recommendations for SC hyoscine butylbromide

Indication	Stat and p.r.n. doses	Initial infusion rate/24h	Common range
Inoperable bowel obstruction with colic[23,24]	20mg	60mg	60–120mg[a]
Death rattle	20mg	20–40mg	20–40mg

a. maximum dose = 300mg/24h.

Hyoscine *hydrobromide* by any route and hyoscine *butylbromide* SC can also be used in other situations where an antimuscarinic may be beneficial, e.g. sialorrhoea.

Despite a plasma halflife of about 8h, the duration of the antisecretory effect after a single dose in *volunteers* is only about 1h (*butylbromide*) and 2h (*hydrobromide*). Thus, hyoscine is best given by CSCI.

In countries such as the USA where hyoscine *butylbromide* is not available, SC glycopyrronium can be substituted, i.e. 200–400microgram stat and p.r.n., and 600–1200microgam/24h by CSCI.[25] Glycopyrronium is the antisecretory drug of choice at some centres in the UK.[26]

References

1 Twycross R *et al.* (2002) *Palliative Care Formulary* (2e). Radcliffe Medical Press, Oxford, pp 1–4.
2 Twycross R *et al.* (2002) *Palliative Care Formulary* (2e). Radcliffe Medical Press, Oxford, pp 219–225.
3 Vecht C *et al.* (1994) Dose-effect relationship of dexamethasone on Karnofsky performance in metastatic brain tumors. A randomized study of doses of 4, 8 and 16 mg per day. *Neurology.* **44:** 675–680.
4 Committee on Safety of Medicines and Medicines Control Agency (1998) Withdrawal of systemic corticosteroids. *Current Problems in Pharmacovigilance.* **24:** 5–7.
5 Twycross R *et al.* (2002) *Palliative Care Formulary* (2e). Radcliffe Medical Press, Oxford, pp 64–67.
6 Foster S *et al.* (1997) Efficacy of lorazepam and haloperidol for rapid tranquilization in the psychiatric emergency room setting. *International Clinical Psychopharmacology* **12:** 175–179.
7 Rey E *et al.* (1999) Pharmacokinetic optimization of benzodiazepines therapy for acute seizures. Focus on delivery routes. *Clinical Pharmacokinetics.* **36:** 409–424.
8 British National Formulary (2001) Drugs used in status epilepticus. *British National Formulary* No. 41. British Medical Association and Royal Pharmaceutical Society of Great Britain, London, p. 234.
9 Treiman D *et al.* (1998) A comparison of four treatments for generalized convulsive status epilepticus. *New England Journal of Medicine.* **339:** 792–798.
10 Peppers M (1996) Benzodiazepines for alcohol withdrawal in the elderly and in patients with liver disease. *Pharmacotherapy.* **16:** 49–57.
11 Chick J (1998) Review: benzodiazepines are more effective than neuroleptics in reducing delirium and seizures in alcohol withdrawal. *Evidence-Based Medicine.* **3:** 11.
12 Twycross R *et al.* (2002) *Palliative Care Formulary* (2e). Radcliffe Medical Press, Oxford, pp 69–70.
13 Twycross R *et al.* (2002) *Palliative Care Formulary* (2e). Radcliffe Medical Press, Oxford, pp 73–74.
14 Wilcock A and Twycross R (1996) Case report: midazolam for intractable hiccup. *Journal of Pain and Symptom Management.* **12:** 59–61.
15 Bauer T *et al.* (1995) Prolonged sedation due to accumulation of conjugated metabolites of midazolam. *Lancet.* **346:** 145–147.
16 Twycross R *et al.* (2002) *Palliative Care Formulary* (2e). Radcliffe Medical Press, Oxford, pp 76–77.

17 Geddes J *et al.* (2000) Atypical antipsychotics in the treatment of schizophrenia: systematic overview and meta-regression analysis. *British Medical Journal.* **321:** 1371–1376.
18 Twycross R *et al.* (2002) *Palliative Care Formulary* (2e). Radcliffe Medical Press, Oxford, pp 80–85.
19 Twycross R *et al.* (2002) *Palliative Care Formulary* (2e). Radcliffe Medical Press, Oxford, pp 339–343.
20 Twycross R *et al.* (2002) *Palliative Care Formulary* (2e). Radcliffe Medical Press, Oxford, pp 4–5.
21 Schuurkes JAJ *et al.* (1986) Stimulation of gastroduodenal motor activity: dopaminergic and cholinergic modulation. *Drug Development Research.* **8:** 233–241.
22 Twycross R *et al.* (2002) *Palliative Care Formulary* (2e). Radcliffe Medical Press, Oxford, pp 5–6, 118–120.
23 DeConno F *et al.* (1991) Continuous subcutaneous infusion of hyoscine butylbromide reduces secretions in patients with gastrointestinal obstruction. *Journal of Pain and Symptom Management.* **6:** 484–486.
24 Baines M (1997) ABC of palliative care: nausea, vomiting and intestinal obstruction. *British Medical Journal.* **315:** 1148–1150.
25 Twycross R *et al.* (2002) *Palliative Care Formulary* (2e). Radcliffe Medical Press, Oxford, pp 287–289.
26 Bennett M *et al.* (2002) Using anti-muscarinic drugs in the management of death rattle: evidence based guidelines for palliative care. *Palliative Medicine.* **16:** 369–374.

PART SIX   **Final thoughts**

As death approaches
When all is said and done
Professional carers have needs too

As death approaches

With increasing weakness, the patient is faced with the fact that death is inevitable and imminent. Support and companionship are of paramount importance at this time.

Weakness is associated both with the need to rest more frequently and with drowsiness. Explanation is essential:

'This often happens in an illness like yours.'   [The doctor understands]

'When the body is short of energy it   [The patient understands]
takes a lot more effort to do even simple
jobs. This means you'll need to rest more
in order to restock your limited energy
supply.'

For the patient who has not yet come to terms with the situation:

'I think a few quiet days in bed are called   [Not destroying hope,
for. If tomorrow or the next day you are   breaking bad news
feeling more energetic, of course you can   gently, giving the
get up but, for the moment, bed is probably   patient permission to let
the best place for you.'   go]

For the spouse and close family:

'This weakness is normal. The cancer is   [The patient is not to
like a parasite and is sapping all his energy.' blame. Also he is not odd
                                               or bad]

'I think the illness is beginning to win.'   [Time is short]

Unless there is a reversible cause, in a progressive disease like cancer, patients probably have a prognosis of only a few days when they become:

- profoundly weak
- bedbound
- semi-comatose
- unable to take tablets or have great difficulty swallowing them
- unable to take more than sips of water.

Although you may feel powerless in the face of rapidly approaching death, patients are generally more realistic. They know you cannot perform a miracle and time is limited. Despite possibly having nothing new to offer:

- continue to visit
- quietly indicate that 'The important thing now is to keep you as comfortable as possible'
- simplify medication: 'Now that your husband is not so well, he can probably manage without so many tablets'
- arrange for medication to be given SL, PR or SC, preferably by CSCI when the patient cannot swallow
- continue to inform the family of the changing situation
  'He is very weak now, but may still live for several days'
  'Although he seems better today, he's still very weak. He could quickly deteriorate and die within a few days'
- control agitation even if it results in sedation
- listen to the nurses.

When all is said and done

Caring for the dying is full of paradoxes. One general practitioner wrote: 'I have looked after several patients who died at home. I still find it extremely harrowing but very rewarding'. Another doctor said to a patient's wife as he left the house: 'I don't know why I keep visiting; I never do anything'. To which the wife replied: 'Oh, Doctor Smith, don't say that! If only you knew the difference your visits make to us'.

Palliative care developed as a reaction to the attitude, spoken or unspoken, that 'there's nothing more that we can do for you', with the inevitable consequence for the patient and family of a sense of abandonment, hopelessness and despair. It was stressed that this was never true, there is always something that can be done. Even so, there are times when the doctor or nurse feels that they have nothing to offer. In this circumstance one is thrown back on who one is as an individual. Sheila Cassidy has illustrated this in a series of sketches (Figures 6.1–6.4).

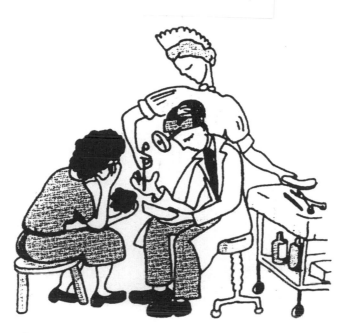

Figure 6.1 This shows the doctor, armed with his competence and his instruments and protected by his aide.[1] (Figures 6.1–6.4 are reproduced with permission.)

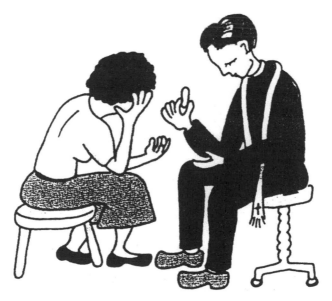

Figure 6.2 A priest performing his sacramental ministry. Here we see him wearing his stole and clerical collar protected by having a role to play and a ritual to perform.[1]

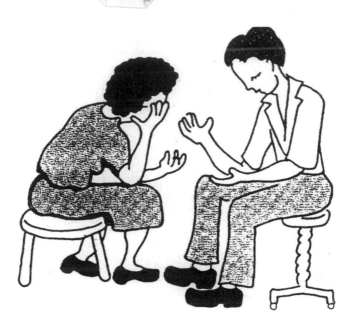

Figure 6.3   A patient meeting with either doctor or clergyman when he has exhausted the physical aspects of his ministry. He is left with his hands empty, but with his resources of counselling still available.[1]

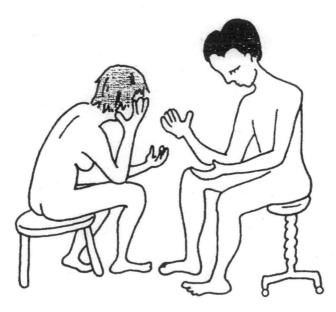

Figure 6.4   Both patient and carer stripped of their resources, present to each other, naked and empty-handed, as two human beings.[1]

> 'Slowly, I learn about the importance of powerlessness.
> I experience it in my own life and I live with it in my work.
> The secret is not to be afraid of it – not to run away.
> The dying know we are not God.
> All they ask is that we do not desert them.'[1]

When there is nothing to offer except ourselves, a belief that life has meaning and purpose helps to sustain the carer. However, to speak glibly of this to a patient who is in despair is cruel. At such times, actions speak louder than words. The essential message is conveyed by what is done:

> 'You matter because you are you.
> You matter to the last moment of your life,
> and we will do all we can
> not only to help you die peacefully,
> but to live until you die.'[2]

> 'Those who have the strength and the love to sit with a dying patient in the silence that goes beyond words will know that this moment is neither frightening nor painful, but a peaceful cessation of the functioning of the body.
>
> Watching a peaceful death of a human being reminds us of a falling star, one of the millions of lights in a vast sky that flares up for a brief moment only to disappear into the endless night forever.'[3]

Professional carers have needs too

Palliative care places many stresses on the professional carer. These include:

- breaking bad news
- coping with the failure of medical cure
- repeated exposure to the death of people with whom we have formed a relationship
- involvement in emotional conflicts
- absorption of anger and grief expressed by patient and families
- role-blurring in multiprofessional teamwork
- personal idealism
- challenges to personal belief systems.

Prerequisites for personal sustenance include:[4]

- feeling loved
- self-esteem
- a body image you accept
- imagination
- being creative
- flexibility
- humour
- compassion
- a capacity to accept mistakes and the ability to correct them
- a readiness to take challenges.

> 'Caring is the result of an ongoing creative process. If creativity is arrested or stopped, caring and hope are not possible. You have to restore creativity in order to restore hope.'[4]

Various strategies help to preserve emotional and physical health and avoid burnout:

- work as a team
    shared decisions and responsibility
    mutual support and respect
- good communications within the team
- good resources and support services
- realistic goals
- be open to receive support from your patients
- adequate off-duty/food/rest
- time for recreation
    hobbies
    spiritual refreshment.

Sometimes it is helpful to have the support of an outside professional counsellor, clinical psychologist or psychotherapist. There are many opportunities for personal growth within the challenges of palliative care. These challenges can be welcomed despite often being painful:

- facing one's own mortality
- facing one's own limitations personally and professionally
- sharing control
- learning to be with patients, not just doing things for them

- facing challenges to one's own beliefs
- dealing honestly with personal emotions, e.g. anger, grief, hurt.

Finally, it is important to remember the rewards of palliative care:

- achieving symptom relief
- facilitating psychological adjustment
- belonging to a supportive team
- time to do things thoroughly
- inspiration from patients and relatives
- personal development.

References

1 Cassidy S (1988) *Sharing the Darkness.* Darton, Longman and Todd, London, pp 61–64.
2 Saunders C. Unpublished talk.
3 Kubler-Ross E (1969) *On Death and Dying.* Tavistock, London.
4 Bild R (1994) Personal communication.

Index